IRON SHIRT CHI KUNG I

*I have come upon Master Chia's Taoist
practice in my old age and find it the most
satisfying and enriching practice of all
those I have encountered in a long life of
seeking and practicing.*

Felix Morrow
Healing Tao Books

IRON SHIRT CHI KUNG I

*Once a Martial Art, Now the Practice
that Strengthens the Internal Organs,
Roots Oneself Solidly, and Unifies
Physical, Mental and Spiritual Health*

MANTAK CHIA

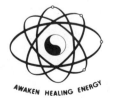

AWAKEN HEALING ENERGY

HEALING TAO BOOKS/Huntington, New York

CONTENTS

The Goal of the Taoist Practice
International Healing Tao Course Offerings
Outline of the Complete System of the Healing Tao
Course Descriptions:
    Introductory Level I: Awaken Healing Light
    Introductory Level II: Development of Internal Power
    Introductory Level III: The Way of Radiant Health
    Intermediate Level:Foundations of Spiritual Practice
    Advance Level:The Realm of Soul and spirit
Healing Tao Books
The International Healing Tao Centers

ACKNOWLEDGMENTS

I thank foremost those Taoist Masters who were kind enough to share their knowledge with me, never imagining it would eventually be taught to Westerners. I acknowledge special thanks to Roberta Prada and Roderick Kettlewell for encouraging the production of this book, for their input on the original manuscript, and for their editing regarding technical procedures.

I thank the many contributors essential to the book's final form: the artist, Juan Li, for many hours spent drawing, making illustrations of the body's internal functions and for the artwork on the cover of the book; Terry Goss for his chapter regarding Breath Alignment which helps tremendously in the practice of Iron Shirt; Larry Short for sharing some of the Tibetan Nui Kung Exercises; Michael Brosnahan for helping to clarify the technical points of structure; Dr. Michael Posner for sharing his view of Chiropractic and Iron Shirt; Gunther Weil, Ph.D., Rylin Malone, and many of my students for their feedback; Jo Ann Cutreria, our secretary, for making so many contacts and working endlessly; Daniel Bobek for long hours at the computer; John-Robert Zielinski for setting up the new computer system and for his interview of Michael Winn; Valerie Meszaros for editing the book, organizing, typing, and revising it on the computer, and proofreading; Helen Stites for proofreading; Adam Sacks, our computer consultant, who assisted in solving computer problems as they arose during the final stages of production; Michael Winn for general editing, and Cathy Umphress for design and paste ups. Special thanks are extended to David Miller for overseeing design and production and to Felix Morrow for his valuable advice and help in editing and producing this book and for agreeing to be the publisher of Healing Tao Books.

Without my mother, my wife, Maneewan, and my son, Max, the book would have been academic—for their gifts, my gratitude and love.

ABOUT MASTER MANTAK CHIA

Master Mantak Chia is the creator of the system known as The Healing Tao and is the Founder and Director of the Healing Tao Center in New York. Since childhood he has been studying the Tao way of life as well as other disciplines. The result of Master Chia's thorough knowledge of Taoism, enhanced by his knowledge of various other systems, is his development of the Healing Tao System, which is now being taught in many cities in the United States, Canada and Europe.

Master Chia was born in Thailand to Chinese parents in 1944, and when he was six years old he learned to "sit and still the mind"—i.e., meditation—from Buddhist monks. While he was a grammar school student, he first learned traditional Thai boxing and then was taught Tai Chi Chuan by Master Lu, who soon introduced him to Aikido, Yoga and more Tai Chi.

Later, when he was a student in Hong Kong excelling in track and field events, a senior classmate, Cheng Sue-Sue, presented him to his first esoteric teacher and most important Taoist Master, Master Yi Eng, and he began his studies of the Taoist way of life. He learned how to pass life-force power from his hands, how to circulate energy through the Microcosmic Orbit, how to open the Six Special Channels, Fusion of the Five Elements, Inner Alchemy, Enlightenment of the Kan and Li, Sealing of the Five Sense Organs, Congress of Heaven and Earth, and Reunion of Man and Heaven. It was Master Yi Eng who authorized Master Chia to teach and heal.

In his early twenties, Mantak Chia studied with Master Meugi in Singapore, who taught him Kundalini and Taoist Yoga and the Buddhist Palm, and he was soon able to get rid of blockages of the flow of life-force energy in his own body as well as in the patients of his Master.

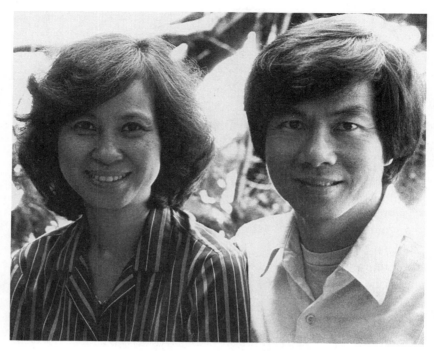
Mantak and Maneewan Chia

In his later twenties, he studied with Master Pan Yu, whose system combined Taoist, Buddhist and Zen teachings, and with Master Cheng Yao-Lun, whose system combined Thai boxing and Kung Fu. From Master Pan Yu he learned about the exchange of the Yin and Yang power between men and women and also the "Steel Body", a technique that keeps the body from decaying. Master Cheng Yao-Lun taught him the secret Shao-Lin Method of Internal Power and the even more secret Iron Shirt methods called "Cleansing the Marrow" and "Renewal of the Tendons".

Then, to better understand the mechanisms behind the healing energy, Master Chia studied Western medical science and anatomy for two years. While pursuing his studies, he managed the Gestetner Company, a manufacturer of office equipment, and became well-acquainted with the technology of offset printing and copying machines.

Using his knowledge of the complete system of Taoism as the foundation, and building onto that with what he learned from his other studies, he developed the Healing Tao System and began teaching it to others. He then trained teachers to assist him, and later established the Natural Healing Center in Thailand. Five years later he decided to move to New York to introduce his system to the West, and in 1979 he opened the Healing Tao Center there. Since then, centers are building in many other locations, including Boston, Philadelphia, Denver, Seattle, San Francisco, Los Angeles, San Diego, Tucson and Toronto, and groups are forming in Europe, in England, Germany, The Netherlands and Switzerland.

Master Chia leads a peaceful life with his wife Maneewan, who teaches Taoist Five Element Nutrition at the New York Center, and their young son. He is a warm, friendly and helpful man, who views himself primarily as a teacher. He uses a word processor when writing his books and is equally at ease with the latest computer technology as he is with esoteric philosophies.

To date he has written and published four Healing Tao Books: in 1983, *Awaken Healing Energy Through the Tao;* in 1984, *Taoist Secrets of Love: Cultivating Male Sexual Energy;* in 1985, *Taoist Ways to Transform Stress into Vitality* and *Chi Self-Massage: The Tao Way of Rejuvenation. Iron Shirt Chi Kung I* is his fifth book.

HOW TO USE THIS BOOK

In the last pages of this book the reader will find descriptions of the courses and workshops offered by our Healing Tao Centers. This material is also, in effect, a comprehensive description of the whole Taoist System. All of my books together will be a composite of this Taoist world-view. Each of my books is thus an exposition of one important part of this system. Each sets forth a method of healing and life-enhancement which can be studied and practiced by itself, if the reader so chooses. However, each of these methods implies the others and is best practiced in combination with the others.

The foundation of all practices in the Taoist System, the Microcosmic Orbit Meditation, is the way to circulate CHI energy throughout the body and is described in my book, *Awaken Healing Energy Through the Tao*. This practice is followed by the meditations of the Inner Smile and the Six Healing Sounds, set forth in my book, *Taoist Ways to Transform Stress into Vitality*. All three meditations are emphasized throughout the Taoist System.

The practices of Iron Shirt Chi Kung are very powerful, and therefore, very effective. To insure that you carry them out properly, prepare yourself first by learning the Microcosmic Orbit Meditation, the Inner Smile and the Six Healing Sounds. These will enable you to identify and eliminate energy blockages that may occur in your Iron Shirt practice during the learning stages.

Second, learn information contained in the chapter in this book on body alignment.

Third, understand the rooting principles.

Fourth, learn the preliminary exercises until you are proficient at them and comfortable with them. This will give you the conditioning you need to proceed comfortably to the postures.

You can use the complete description of each posture during your learning. The shorter description of each posture is meant as a guide during your practice.

Lastly, we offer to you a suggested practice timetable, although it is not necessary for you to follow it exactly. Use it merely as a guideline for adjusting your own schedule.

As you read the information provided in this book and become aware of concepts not contained in Western thought, you will deepen your understanding of the relevancy of these practices to your physical, emotional and spiritual advancement.

Mantak Chia

A WORD OF CAUTION

The book does not give any diagnoses or suggestions for medication. It does provide a means to increase your strength and good health in order to overcome imbalances in your system. For people who have high blood pressure, heart disease, or a generally weak condition, proceed slowly in your practice of packing. If there is illness, a medical doctor should be consulted.

1. GENERAL INTRODUCTION

A. *The Healing Tao System and Iron Shirt Chi Kung*

In addition to the more popularly known martial arts disciplines of Kung Fu and Tai Chi, the Healing Tao System includes health practices, healing arts, the development of a state of mindfulness, and the management of vital energy (CHI). The martial arts aspect of this training, the practice of Iron Shirt, develops a highly refined moral and spiritual awareness.

The goal of the Healing Tao System is to keep our physical bodies in good condition in the physical plane in order to build and store more CHI energy for further use in the higher level of the spiritual plane. (Figure 1–1)

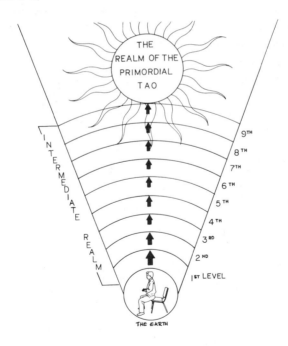

FIGURE 1-1

The Realm of the Primordial Tao

In the spiritual plane, the aim is to develop the immortal fetus. The immortal fetus is developed in two stages. The first stage is concerned with overcoming reincarnation. The next stage develops and educates the immortal fetus to become a full-grown immortal spirit.

Iron Shirt is one of the most important exercises of the physical plane because through its practice one learns rootedness to Mother Earth energy, a phenomenon intrinsic to the spiritual plane. (Figure 1–2)

One may compare the foundation, or rootedness, of the physical body to an Earth Control Tower, vital to the travel of a space shuttle

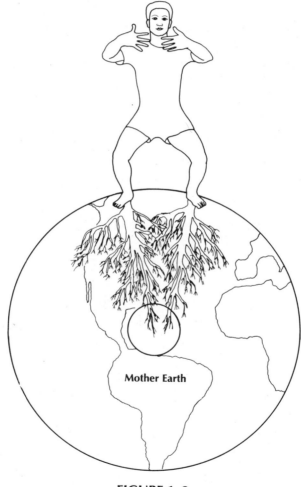

Mother Earth

FIGURE 1–2

Rootedness to Mother Earth Energy

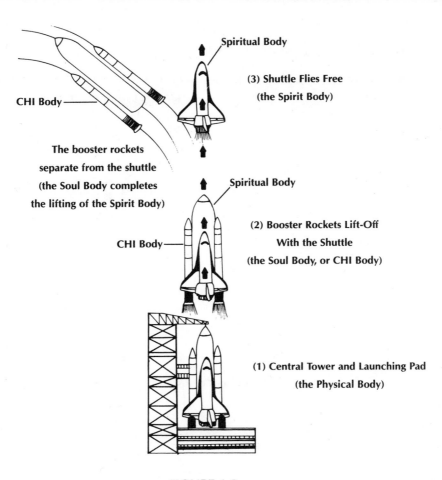

FIGURE 1-3

Launching of the Spiritual Body

in space. (Figure 1–3) To boost the space shuttle, the spirit, into space the Earth Control Tower requires a booster rocket, the soul or energy body, which is guided by an inner compass and computer, the pineal gland. The Earth Control Tower, in the form of our physical body developed during the practice of Iron Shirt, becomes a storage place for fuel: CHI (our life-force energy) and our creative (or sexual) energy. Here our fuel awaits transformation into another kind of energy: spiritual energy. As we learn how to develop an immortal spirit compass and computer by opening the pineal gland which will guide us back to Earth to complete the unfinished job of development here, we must maintain our foundation, or rootedness, to the Earth. (Figure 1–4) Thus we are able to return to Earth, refuel and resume our space travel to our destination until, eventually, we are able to discard the earthly base entirely.

FIGURE 1-4

Rootedness

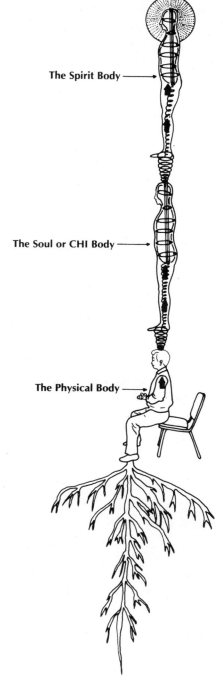

The Spirit Body

The Soul or CHI Body

The Physical Body

1. Iron Shirt Chi Kung, an Ancient Kung Fu Practice

a. The Bolin Period (the Time of Kung Fu Fighters)

Kung Fu was used in China long before the advent of firearms. During the Bolin Period, approximately 1000 b.c., training in the various spiritual/martial arts was very intense. It is said that at the time one-tenth the population of China was involved in some sort of Kung Fu.

In ancient Kung Fu practice, training began in very early youth. One first worked to develop internal power (inner strength through organ exercise), a venture that could take as long as ten years. Thereafter, one might have to throw a straight punch 1,000 times a day for a period lasting from three to five years. One might be instructed to strike the top of a water-well with the flat of his palm 1,000 times a day for five to ten years, or "until the water leapt out of the well".

Iron Shirt Chi Kung, a method of Kung Fu, was learned as a protective training, providing internal power by the practice of simple external techniques. The practitioner was guarded against the effects of blows to his vital organs and glands, the primary sources for the production of life-force energy (CHI). The word CHI means air. Kung means discipline: one who puts time into practice. Therefore, Chi Kung means "to practice the process of breathing to increase CHI pressure (life-force pressure)".

A thousand times a day internal power was cultivated until it could be felt flowing out of the hands. With weights tied to the legs, the practitioner ran and jumped in prescribed ways for over three hours a day until, eventually, he could jump easily to great heights and, at the same time, further develop his internal power. Only after these exercises were mastered were actual fighting techniques taught.

The importance of the development of internal power in martial arts training may be compared to the effect of being struck by a steel rod as opposed to one that is made of soft plastic. The Chi Kung practitioner of old practiced one punch for years until he could feel the power go out of the lower part of his hand, while the rest of his body seemed as though made of steel. There were many other benefits as well, e.g., internal power improved general health and is claimed to have maintained youthfulness.

b. Iron Shirt Helps to Perfect Mental Faculties

Chi Kung also helped to perfect mental faculties, enabling the practitioner to have knowledge of many things. One reads that during the Bolin period, there were eight "immortals" who spent most of their lives in such practice and developed extraordinary abilities. They could predict the future and see into the past. They are said to have been capable of space travel and of clairvoyance and clairaudience. It is also said that during that period, many people had at least some such powers, a result of widespread Kung Fu practice. Some sources attempt to explain this by claiming there must have been a general universal reservoir of power, far greater than is now available, from which the more capable practitioners could draw.

c. The Age of Gunpowder

After the invention of gunpowder and the subsequent elaboration of firearms, men no longer felt the need to spend a decade or more of their lives learning skills that no longer seemed practical. A man could now defend himself, or cause great damage at a great distance from his objective, with weapons. (Figure 1–5) Contact fighting became a thing of the past, and much of the associated knowledge that was useful to man was lost with it.

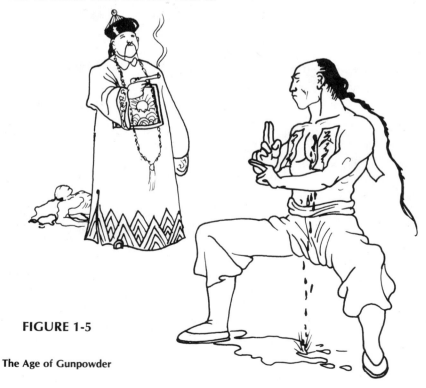

FIGURE 1-5

The Age of Gunpowder

Today, however, with the recent revolt against the depersonalizing and unhealthy effects of a technology of monstrous proportions, there has been a revival of interest in the simpler ways of life. Thus, Kung Fu is again in the limelight. Kung Fu has been called a way of perfecting the inner self.

2. Creating CHI (Life-Force) Pressure

Chi Kung may be thought of as internal aerobics. CHI, as an aerobic energy involving air, steam, and pressure, presses out and circulates to protect the human body. One can compare the internal pressure created by CHI to the force of air in a tire which is sufficient to keep the tire inflated and maintain a cushion between the car and the road. (Figure 1–6)

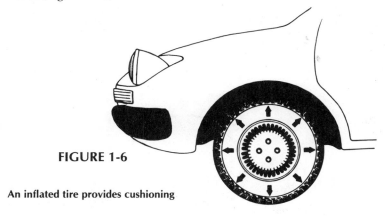

FIGURE 1-6

An inflated tire provides cushioning

a. The Breath of Life, CHI Pressure

Breathing is the most important part of our lives. We can go without food for months, or without water for days, but we can go without air for only a few minutes.

In practicing Iron Shirt, we use our breath to maximum advantage. We can actually increase our vital energy, strengthen our organs, and promote self-healing by increasing the CHI pressure (pounds per square inch) in the organs and cavity of the body. The circulatory system, the lymphatic system, the nervous system, and the endocrine glands will be activated, and blood, spinal fluid and hormones will flow more easily so that the heart will not have to work hard.

b. The Origin of Iron Shirt Breathing

Taoists believe that while we are in the womb, we use Iron Shirt Packing Breathing. Before birth, the infant does not use the lungs and nose to breathe. The CHI (life-force) enters through the umbilical cord to the navel (Figure 1–7), down to the perineum, up the sacrum to the spinal cord to the head, forehead, and down the front from the tongue (Taoists believe the fetus always holds the tongue on the palate) to the throat, heart, abdomen and navel centers in the abdominal area where the CHI pressure can be used. You will recognize this as the path of the Microcosmic Orbit (described more fully in Chapter 2).

At birth, we begin to use lung breathing and generate our own energy rather than use the internal source of energy. To begin with, the lungs are not strong. The abdomen, closer to our original source of energy in the navel, has more CHI pressure. It assists the lungs in breathing by pulling down on the diaphragm so that the lower portion of the lungs fills with air, initiating inhalation. In this way, the

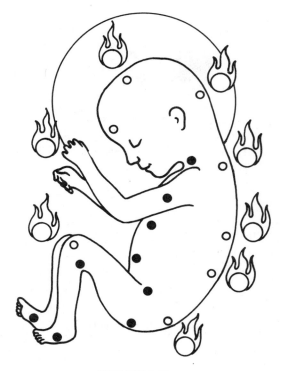

FIGURE 1-7

**In an unborn infant, the CHI (life-force)
enters through the umbilical cord to the navel**

lungs use less energy, but take in more life-force (oxygen). As children, we still use abdominal CHI pressure energy.

One can see the effects of reduced CHI pressure with age. In older people the prenatal life-force (CHI) is drained out from the navel and kidney areas. Gradually CHI pressure is lost, creating an energy imbalance: when the pressure is low, the fluid flow in the entire system slows down. As a result, at the times when our energy becomes too hot, it will move up and congest the chest and head. Cold energy will move down through the sexual organs and leak out. Gradually, we lose CHI pressure. We begin to lose the habit of abdominal breathing. The lungs are left alone to do chest breathing.

This is inefficient. It requires greater energy to expand the rib cage, which action fills only the upper third of the lungs. Scientists have affirmed that we use only one-third of our vital capacity (lung capacity) for breathing. This method of breathing actually expends more energy than it creates. Yielding to the external pressure, we collapse inside. With abdominal breathing, we can expand the amount of pressure exerted on the organs and voluntarily compress them so that they will strengthen upon release.

B. Why Put on Your Iron Shirt?

1. Internal Management

Many of the physical changes associated with Kung Fu come through management of the internal organs and endocrine glands.

In Kung Fu, a person's life-force is said to depend primarily upon the endocrine glands, or sexual hormones. It is very likely that this was deduced from the following observations.

Consider what happens when someone is deprived of a fully functional endocrine system. A male is radically altered when his testes, part of the endocrine system in males, are eliminated, and more so when this is done before puberty. Such characteristics as weak musculature and feminine fat distribution develop. Depending upon the time in life in which he was so mutilated, he might also lack such secondary male characteristics as a deep voice, facial hair and sexual drive. Male and female castrates have been well documented to have shortened life spans.

With Iron Shirt Chi Kung, one is able to increase the flow of hormones produced by the endocrine glands, building up the immune system and giving a general sense of well-being. The sexual (creative) energy produced as a result is another source of CHI energy which may later be transformed into spiritual energy.

Integral to Iron Shirt are the organs' exercises which clean and strengthen the organs. Strong, detoxified organs are important to modern life. Iron Shirt practice will strengthen; help to clean out the toxins, waste materials and sediment in the organs; and convert the fat stored in layers or sheaths of connective tissue (fasciae) in the body into CHI energy. The CHI is subsequently stored in the fasciae layers where it works like a cushion to protect the organs. As previously mentioned, this process may be compared to a tire which, when inflated with air, can sustain tremendous weight. CHI which has been stored in such a way then becomes available for transformation to a higher quality energy that can nourish the soul and spirit.

In the practice of Iron Shirt, we put more emphasis on the fasciae connective tissues, organs, tendons, bones and bone marrow and less emphasis on muscle development.

a. CHI, the Fasciae, Organs and Bones

The body may be conceived as consisting of three layers: (a) the innermost which is made up of the internal organs that produce CHI; (b) a layer consisting of fasciae, bones and tendons; and (c) the muscles, which constitute the bulk of the body. CHI, after being developed in the internal organs, is then distributed throughout the fasciae. It is with the fasciae that Iron Shirt I is primarily concerned.

(1) The Fasciae

Each organ has a fascia layer covering it. (Figure 1–8) In the heart this layer is called the pericardium; in the lung it is called the pleura. The fasciae which cover the stomach, liver and kidneys have protective, connective, regenerative and nourishing properties. They act as energizing chambers for the organs.

In Heller work and Rolfing massaging techniques, the fasciae is dealt with from the outside in. The art of Rolfing involves the freeing

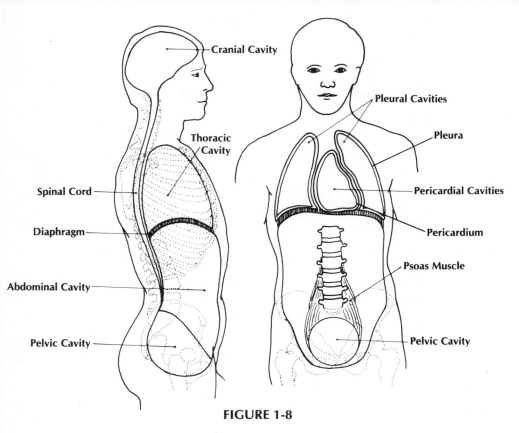

FIGURE 1-8

Each organ has a fascia layer covering its cavity

of areas of fasciae that have become stuck together through trauma, infection or chronic muscular tensions. Iron Shirt works from the inner layer of fascia out. (Figure 1–9) The intent is to allow for a free flowing energy in the body and to enable psychological insight into events long harbored in restricted musculature.

The fasciae are extremely important in the practice of Iron Shirt because, as the most pervasive tissues in the body, they are believed to be the means whereby CHI is distributed along acupuncture routes. Research has shown that the least resistance to the flow of bioelectric energy in the body occurs between the fascial sheaths, and that when these routes have been charted, they have been found to correspond to the classical acupuncture channels.

(2) Iron Shirt Strengthens and Protects the Organs

When we pack and wrap the organs with CHI pressure, we start

29

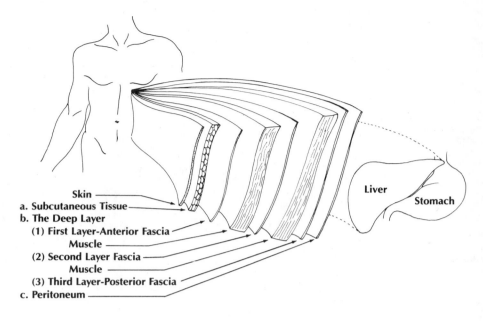

Skin
a. Subcutaneous Tissue
b. The Deep Layer
    (1) First Layer-Anterior Fascia
           Muscle
    (2) Second Layer Fascia
           Muscle
    (3) Third Layer-Posterior Fascia
c. Peritoneum

Liver

Stomach

FIGURE 1-9

Fasciae Layers

to strengthen the organs. The fasciae layers covering the organs, when filled with CHI pressure, will act as energizers to the organs. Extra CHI pressure will escape to the abdominal fascia layer, fill the abdominal cavity with CHI pressure, act as a protector to the organs and permit the CHI to flow more easily. When the abdominal cavity fills with CHI pressure, the CHI pressure will start to fill in the deep fasciae and, finally, fill in the outer layer, acting as a triple layer of cushion of CHI pressure to pack and protect all of the organs, muscles and vital glands.

To better understand how CHI, the fasciae and the organs relate to one another, picture an egg residing inside a balloon filled with air, residing inside another air-filled balloon, both of which reside inside one more air-filled balloon. (Figure 1–10) An egg is normally quite vulnerable, but inside a blown-up balloon, it is cushioned against blows. Inside a triple layer of balloons, we see that the egg has even greater protection. You can throw and kick these three layers of balloons and the egg will remain unharmed. CHI and the fasciae act in the same way to protect the fragile organs. The fasciae are elastic and protective

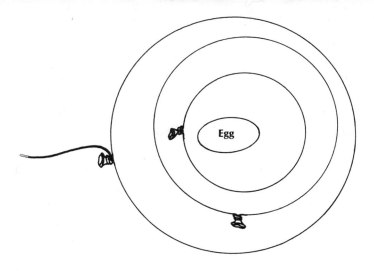

FIGURE 1-10

Balloons containing an egg

like balloons, and the CHI, expanding as the air expands within the ballons, creates internal pressure. (Figure 1–11)

When CHI pressure is reduced by sickness or a weakened state, the organs become cramped because they yield and become compressed by pressures external to them.

Most people, when hit in the abdomen, will fall down or, if they are so unlucky as to have the vital organs hit, are seriously injured in the vital organs. When the vital organs are injured, life can be endan-

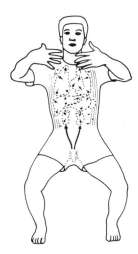

FIGURE 1-11

Pack the CHI into the organs and fasciae layers to protect the organs   31

gered. With this practice of building layers of protection, you will greatly reduce the risk of unexpected injury and in many instances might help to save your life.

From the fasciae, Iron Shirt extends to involve the bones and tendons and, finally, the muscles.

(3) Burn Out Fat and Store CHI in the Organs

Food (nutrition) that is taken into the body but is not required by the body is turned into fat and stored in the outer layers of fasciae. This fat will greatly reduce the flow of CHI. The Iron Shirt Packing Process will help to pack and squeeze the fat, transforming it into energy to be stored in the fascial covers of the organs for use whenever needed. When CHI pressure occupies the fascial layers, the fat cannot be stored there. Therefore, the body becomes trained to convert fat into CHI energy for storage in the fascial layers.

(4) The Structure of the Bones

When the fasciae are filled with CHI, the tendons are strengthened and the bones hold together as one structural piece. When the fasciae are weak, the muscles are weakened and the bone structure will not hold together. Similarly, when the muscles are weak, both the fasciae and the tendons are weak. When muscles are not used, they diminish in size and strength as do the fasciae which contain them and the tendons upon which they pull when activated.

There is a constant turnover of most of the cells of the body and replacements are governed by ongoing needs. It has been demonstrated that during prolonged periods of weightlessness in outer space, the constitution of bones is not as dense as it is on the surface of the Earth where the greater stresses of gravity signal heavier bone growth. When we are young, our bones are filled with marrow. (Figure 1–12) When we become adults, the bones gradually hollow out, filling with fat and producing less blood cells, until they become brittle and susceptible to fracture. Iron Shirt Chi Kung is primarily designed to gradually reabsorb the CHI life-force back into the bones, which can be transformed into bone marrow to strengthen the bone structure.

b. CHI Pressure and Meditation Increases Circulation while Reducing the Heart's Work

As mentioned, we must learn again to use the abdomen to aid in breathing and to help increase the circulation. The abdominal area

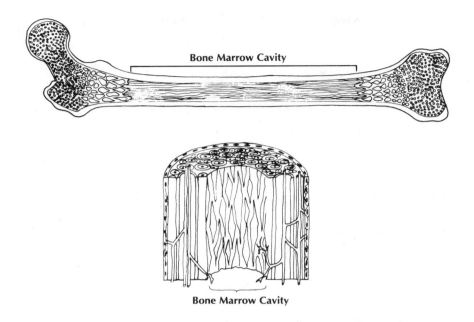

Bone Marrow Cavity

Bone Marrow Cavity

FIGURE 1-12

When we are young, our bones are filled with red marrow

accounts for two-thirds of the blood supply that flows through the liver, kidneys, stomach and spleen. When one knows how to pack and release, the abdomen will act like the most efficient heart you could ever have. In Iron Shirt Chi Kung Packing Process Breathing, by limiting the space of the abdomen and increasing the pounds of pressure per square inch, all the organs in the abdominal area will be packed in a very small space. This will expel all the toxins and sediment which have accumulated in these organs. The diaphragm will pull down to create a vacuum in the lower part of the lungs, filling the lower lobes first, and extending to the whole lungs. This gives a longer, deeper breath which will furnish sufficient time and quantity of oxygen to cleanse the body of waste materials, sediment and toxins.

Our systems rely entirely upon CHI pressure to move the fluids. Increased pressure in the abdominal cavity will help to increase the CHI pressure in order to move CHI, blood and lymph fluids. (Figure

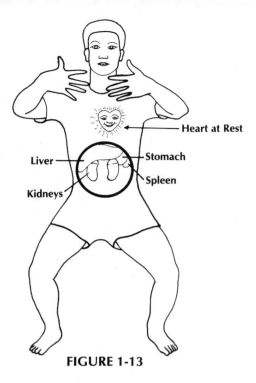

Liver

Heart at Rest

Stomach

Spleen

Kidneys

FIGURE 1-13

Compressing the organs, thereby creating a pressure in the abdomen, can cause the abdomen to pump like a heart, moving fluids through the system

1–13) When the new blood is released, oxygen and nutrition will enter into the organs. With this practice, you will gradually increase the flow of the circulatory and lymph systems and, in return, will greatly reduce the work of the heart. As you gradually increase your vital capacity by learning how to pack air into the organs, thereby creating the cushion, or CHI pressure, to protect and strengthen them, the heart will have to work with progressively less effort, and circulation will increase. The vital energy thus conserved can be used to enrich our spiritual and creative lives.

Our goal, then, is to increase the organ and abdominal pressure so that the CHI presses outward on the fasciae layers from inside. To do this, you will learn Packing Process Breathing to increase the pressure of CHI in the organs and abdomen. When this pressure is released, the fasciae expand as do the organs.

CHI circulation meditation affords a means of generating and directing far more CHI than would ordinarily be available without causing pressure on the heart. Meditation increases circulation and the production of lymphocytes without affecting blood pressure the way running and western aerobic exercises do. Once you have practiced CHI circulation meditation by learning the Microcosmic Orbit, you will understand that the energy made use of in Iron Shirt travels very much along the same route of the Microcosmic Orbit, but is found to be expressed differently in each of the channels. As the CHI flows more freely throughout the entire body, the experience takes on new dimensions.

c. Preventing Energy Leakage

The Taoists believe that CHI can be transformed into anything in our body. Certainly, the energy we channel in the body has a generative effect. Therefore, an important function of Iron Shirt is to learn how to create space in the body to store CHI energy and how to prevent energy leakage. Energy is dispersed and scattered in the average person, escaping out daily through various openings in the body. Iron Shirt teaches the practitioner how to seal these openings. A process is then learned to direct this conserved energy to the navel region, there to be packed and condensed into an energy ball (Figure 1–14) which can be directed to any part of the body or, in later practice, to build an energy body to boost the spirit to a higher plane.

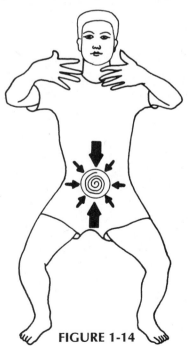

FIGURE 1-14

Concentrating Energy Into an Energy Ball

2. Iron Shirt Prolongs Life

Long life and happiness have been pursued by people for centuries, and the search still continues. However, even with the added impetus of all that modern science and technology can offer, little real, if any, progress has been made that is in the common domain.

It is currently believed by many here in the West that daily physical exercise helps to stave off aging. However, statistically, athletes do not live longer nor seem to be appreciably healthier for their efforts. In fact, as the effects of aging impede them more and more, many of them become subject to depression. They are no longer able to compete successfully. In order to do more strenuous exercises, parts of the body must be changed. Also, there seems to be some basis for thinking that certain situations, such as the stress of competetive athletics or the use of drugs, may contribute to premature aging (discounting injuries that are sustained in more violent pursuits). A Taoist might comment that this is so because in accenting the physical, the spiritual was neglected, as well as the mind, the nervous system and the internal vital circuits.

Man's life span has been prolonged by science and technology. However, more often than not, the added life span can be of a low enough quality that it does not seem to be of great benefit.

The old Taoist sages say that in ancient times, men lived from 500 to 1,000 years. Modern society emphasizes material aspects of life whereas the ancient Taoists sought a balance of the material with the spiritual. The Taoist and Yogic approaches describe an "inner world" which man can develop and cultivate that is reflected in his "outer world". There is an old Taoist saying, "Living one hundred years is common. Life is in my hands, not in the hands of a Universal Being." It might be that this positive statement is derived from a genuine knowledge of how to prolong life in such a way that it is also vital and satisfying.

The Taoist System is very precise in the matter of building CHI, guiding it and finally developing skills to make the best use of it. To attempt to hasten the process by skipping steps is to end with nothing or to create complications such as irregular heartbeat, chest congestion, headache, pain in the heart, chest or back, which result from not knowing how to guide the energy.

3. Summary of the Benefits of Iron Shirt Chi Kung Training

In summary, Iron Shirt Chi Kung I training is divided into three levels: physical, emotional and spiritual.

a. On the physical level, one learns how to (1) align structurally to strengthen and alter a weak structure into a strong structure so that CHI can flow easily throughout the body and provide room for organs to grow within the body's structure; (2) develop a CHI Belt, the major connection of the upper and lower energy channels, without which proper structural alignment and CHI energy will be lost; (3) detoxify and exercise the organs and glands in order to charge and pack the CHI in them, to serve as cushioning to surround and protect them, and to fill the cavity of the body with CHI pressure; (4) increase CHI storage between the fasciae sheets; open the fasciae to serve as CHI storage areas of the body, replacing fat previously stored there; understand the function of the fasciae layers as cushions around the body which protect the vital organs; (5) root down to the earth, sink down and become one with the earth, to be able to pass the outside force down to earth through the structure without obstruction, and to pump the earth force up into the structure and counteract outside forces with the assistance of the earth; (6) generate an easily flowing CHI through the meridians of the body, and transform CHI to a higher "octane" to serve as the nourishment of the soul and spirit body.

b. On the emotional level, or soul level, one learns how to (1) condense the CHI into a controllable mass of energy, transforming and moving the CHI by changing negative energy into positive energy; (2) condense life-force CHI into a ball. This is one of the most important functions of the Iron Shirt Chi Kung practice since it enables one to control his CHI so that the CHI will not scatter around the body and leak out of the system. Condensed CHI will stay together and have more condensed power to be used as a person desires. When you are well-trained in condensing the CHI energy into a ball, by physically moving the abdomen up and down, or left and right, you will be able to move the ball. In later practice, you will be able to use your mind to move the ball and direct it through channels in your body, always returning it to the navel. In the higher level, the condensed CHI becomes a light ball, like a glowing pearl, which develops into the energy body, serving as a booster rocket to boost the spirit or space body into orbit.

c. On the spiritual level, Iron Shirt CHI Kung condenses, strengthens and creates more CHI, thereby laying the groundwork for a spiritual foundation (rootedness) which serves the later part of the system. Previously referred to as an Earth Control Tower, this foundation will direct the spirit in its journey through space where preparations are made for life after death.

C. Iron Shirt Chi Kung Exercises

The Iron Shirt exercises introduced here are primarily concerned with the fasciae and bone structure as well as with some tendons.

These eight exercises (namely, Embracing the Tree, the Yin and Yang Positions of Holding the Golden Urn, the Golden Turtle Immersing in Water (Yang Position), the Water Buffalo Emerging From the Water (Yin Position), The Golden Phoenix Washes Its Feathers, the Iron Bridge and the Iron Bar), condensed from forty-nine postures, are very precise in developing the most vital energy routes. There are many exercises known that will serve this purpose; however, by doing the eight exercises and the structural alignment exercises described in this book, you will derive as much benefit as you would from a much wider selection of positions and movements. These exercises develop CHI flow and strengthen fasciae, tendons, bones and muscles. In the tradition of Taoist Esoteric Yoga, it is said that (a) CHI moves the blood (and the heart works less); (b) blood moves muscles; (c) muscles move tendons, and (d) tendons move the bones to which they are attached.

Iron Shirt strengthens muscles, tendons and bones by subjecting them directly and gradually to increasing stress. It is a well-rounded approach which offers, as an additional benefit, a means of releasing long held areas of tension. This often reflects in a general sense of well-being, of self-assurance and ease, along with better posture.

Many of my students report that Iron Shirt has enabled them to achieve a deep sense of feeling grounded and centered. Others suddenly discover that their hands and feet are no longer cold.

There is another advantage to Iron Shirt. The pneumatic effect joins what would otherwise be separate members of your body into one continuous unit. This produces a tremendous increase in mechanical advantage that increases geometrically as this work progresses.

The Healing Tao System offers many types of practices, many of which can be practiced individually. However, it is most beneficial to the practitioner to realize that all are interrelated and practicing them together will bring the best results. If one attempts to practice Tai Chi Chuan, for example, before having first cultivated internal energy through Iron Shirt, it might be compared to entering high school without having learned the alphabet.

Iron Shirt Chi Kung is the foundation of Tai Chi which uses structural alignment as a basis for exercise. Many people have the wrong idea about Tai Chi. When the energy is felt in the Tai Chi movements, the practitioner wants to move the energy. However, the moving form of Tai Chi occupies the mind with many things other than moving the energy. The more the practitioner moves his form, the busier his mind, making him less aware of the subtle energy that can be felt within himself. In other words, the simpler one keeps the activity of the mind, the better one can feel his inner workings. Iron Shirt uses the mind to guide the CHI flow in a static position. If you train in the methods of Iron Shirt first, you learn well how to move the CHI. Then when you practice Tai Chi, it is easier to move the CHI while practicing the moving forms. In the Healing Tao System, we require students to learn the Microcosmic Orbit, Iron Shirt Chi Kung, and then Tai Chi. Therefore, the structural rooting and energy discharge and control that is learned in Iron Shirt can be transferred into the Tai Chi form. It should also be noted that to practice Tai Chi Chuan properly, it is necessary that your meditation practice take you at least to the levels in the Healing Tao System of Fusion of the Five Elements or to Lesser Enlightenment Kan and Li.

Since the basic approaches of the Microcosmic Orbit, Iron Shirt Chi Kung, Seminal or Ovarian Kung Fu, and Tai Chi Chi Kung deal with some aspect of coaxing energy out of the deepest and outermost reaches of the body, it is wise for the practitioner who is interested in developing fully his physical, emotional and spiritual potential to consider the Healing Tao System in its entirety.

D. Three Levels of Iron Shirt

This first Iron Shirt book is concerned with the first level of Iron Shirt, Iron Shirt Chi Kung I, in which, through internal organs exercises, the fasciae (the connecting tissue which cover the organs and glands) are energized.

The second book, Iron Shirt Chi Kung II, deals with tendon exercises, known since olden times as "Changing the Tendons". This practice utilizes the mind and heart to direct, stretch and grow the tendons.

Iron Shirt Chi Kung III, the third book in this series, works on bone structure and increases the bone marrow. This procedure, known by the ancient Taoists as "Cleansing the Marrow", is used to clear out fat stored in the hollow bone and absorb the creative power (sexual energy) into the bone to rebuild the bone marrow. Bones are the major blood builders, including the white blood cells necessary to the body's defense mechanisms.

2. INITIAL PREPARATIONS

A. *Iron Shirt Breathing and Relaxation*

You must not use force in any of these procedures. These exercises depend very much upon mind control and relaxation. In doing the chin press, which is accomplished by pressing the chin down to the chest and pushing out C–7, the chest must remain relaxed if you are not to develop chest pain and congestion and if you are to avoid difficulty in breathing. Practice the relaxation of the Inner Smile and run your Microcosmic Orbit (described briefly in this Chapter and more fully in the book, *Awaken Healing Energy Through the Tao.*) If you find yourself shaking and jerking about, just simply let it all happen. It is a refreshing experience.

In a standing or walking position, you can stroke your chest with your palms from top to bottom from nine to eighteen times to relieve any congestion that might have accumulated there. Burp, if the need arises. If you begin to salivate copiously, tighten your neck muscles, press your chin to your chest, "smile down" through all of your organs and then put your tongue to your palate and, using force, swallow saliva so that you feel as though you have indeed swallowed all the way down to your navel. Concentrate there until you can feel your navel grow warm.

Practice the Iron Shirt Chi Kung breathing twice per day only during your first week of practice and three times per day in the following week. By the second to fourth week, you can increase six to nine times and increase the length of time in Packing Breathing.

1. Abdominal and Reverse Breathing (Energizer Breathing)

Those who have not been trained in Chi Kung, Yoga or any other breathing exercise will be tense and will use very shallow, short breaths, uilizing only one-third of the lungs. This causes loss of CHI pressure in the abdominal cavity. With practice, proper breathing is accomplished.

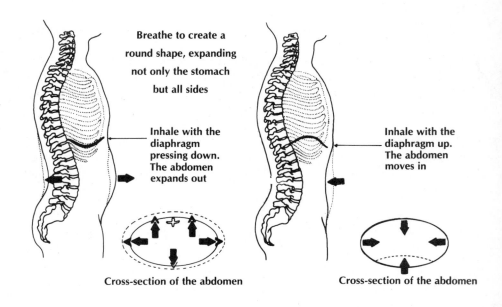

Breathe to create a round shape, expanding not only the stomach but all sides

Inhale with the diaphragm pressing down. The abdomen expands out

Inhale with the diaphragm up. The abdomen moves in

Cross-section of the abdomen

Cross-section of the abdomen

(a) Abdominal Breathing

(b) Reverse Breathing

FIGURE 2-1

Iron Shirt breathing combines various types of breathing. First, abdominal breathing is practiced to energize and loosen the fascial layers of the body. When the breath is harmonized, CHI is sent down to the navel. At this time, reverse breathing is initiated. Abdominal and reverse breathing are the two basic ways of breath training. Practiced together, they are known as Energizer Breathing, but have also been called "Breath of Fire" or "Bellows Breathing".

Abdominal and reverse breathing are caused by the up and down movement of the thoracic diaphragm. (Figure 2–1 (a) and (b)) During abdominal breathing, the diaphragm lowers and forces the vital organs, especially the adrenal glands, to compress downward, allowing the lower lobes of the lungs to fill with air, and forcing the abdomen to protrude. The chest and the sternum sink, which presses and activates the thymus gland. Upon exhalation, the stomach returns to a flatter shape and the other vital organs return to their original size and shape. In reverse breathing, on inhalation we flatten the stomach, push the organs and diaphragm up, and allow air to fill the whole lungs. As your practice develops, you will be able to maintain a lowered diaphragm during reverse breathing, thereby lowering and compressing the organs. Upon exhaling, we fill the abdomen out. The motions thus created massage the vital organs to a certain extent. It is to reverse breathing that "Packing" Breathing is added.

a. Practice Abdominal Breathing (Figure 2–1(a))

(1) To practice abdominal breathing, keep the chest very relaxed. This may be difficult at first, but it is important. Begin by breathing in, drawing the air into the abdomen.

(2) Make the chest hollow and drop the diaphragm down. (Figure 2–2(a)) Pressure is felt inside the abdomen which will begin to protrude on all sides in a rounded shape. Do not expand the stomach only. With the diaphragm lowered and the abdomen filled with air, the inches of spacing containing the abdominal organs are minimized. (Figure 2–2(b))

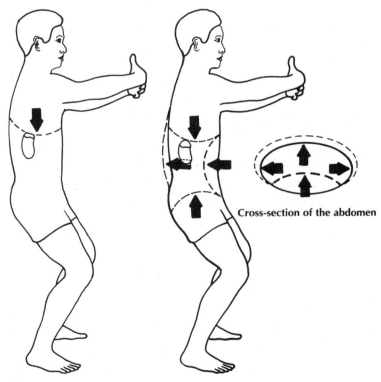

Cross-section of the abdomen

(a) The Diaphragm Pressing Down
on the Adrenals and Kidneys

(b) The Diaphragm, Abdominal Wall and
Perineum Pressing into the Abdomen

FIGURE 2-2

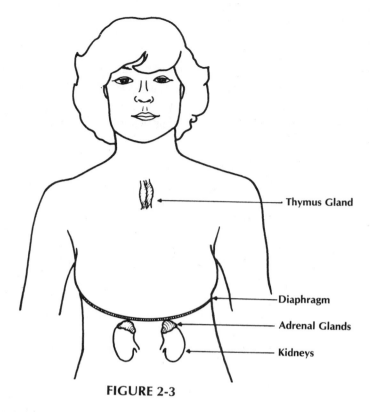

Thymus Gland

Diaphragm

Adrenal Glands

Kidneys

FIGURE 2-3

When the diaphragm presses down on the adrenal glands, the sternum sinks
This activates the thymus gland

(3) Hold your breath for a moment and exhale, flatten the stomach to the spine and feel the perineum (the region between the genital organs and the rectum) flood with the pressure. Pull the sexual organs up. The chest and the sternum sink, pressing and activating the thymus gland. (Figure 2–3) Do not use force. It is enough to feel a slight pull and flattening of the chest.

(4) Inhale and relax, maintaining a dropped diaphragm, and feel the air expand on all sides of the abdomen (not only the front) like a round ball. Exhale and feel the pull of the sexual organs.

(5) With each inhalation and exhalation counting as one set, practice each set nine, eighteen, and then 36 times. Abdominal breathing, as the initiation of what is called "Energizer Breathing", is used throughout all the exercises as a pre-exercise to Packing Process Breathing. It is also used after packing process breathing to regulate the breath.

(6) If you find that your diaphragm becomes tight and pushed up into the rib cage, rub the diaphragm with both hands using the fingers to gently work the diaphragm so that it will drop down out of the rib area into a relaxed position. (Figure 2–4) Tightness in the abdominal area is one of the main causes of breathing problems. Abdominal massage will help to relieve the tightness of the diaphragm. Use your fingers to lightly massage the abdomen in the navel area until you feel the tightness ease. This will greatly improve your deep breathing.

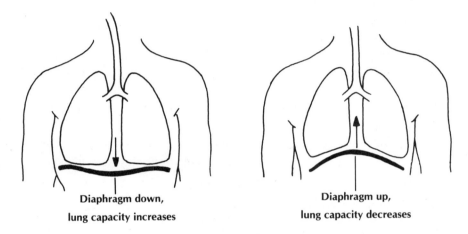

Diaphragm down,
lung capacity increases

Diaphragm up,
lung capacity decreases

FIGURE 2-4

Front View of the Diaphragm

b. Practice Reverse Breathing (Figure 2–1(b))

Tight muscles in the chest can be a problem, and so it is important to relax. It is not the muscles but this relaxation which holds the CHI packed inside. Moreover, using and training the mind to direct and condense the CHI are the ultimate goals of Iron Shirt training.

As you begin to inhale for reverse breathing, the organs and diaphragm are pushed up as the air fills the entire lungs. As your practice develops, you will be able to control the diaphragm and organs, maintaining them in a lowered position.

Reverse breathing, as the preparation for Packing Process Breathing, also takes place in the lower abdomen and should be practiced in conjunction with abdominal breathing. Draw air into the abdomen while contracting the muscles in the front of the abdomen. Begin with abdominal breathing, and follow with reverse breathing.

(1) Practice abdominal breathing six times. Upon the last exhalation, flatten the stomach. Maintain the flattened stomach and begin reverse breathing upon inhalation. Feel the abdomen flatten even more, as if it were approaching the spine and feel the perineum flood with a pressure. Pull the sexual organs up and, at the same time, try to lower the diaphragm so that you are pushing down on the organs. Try not to let the diaphragm push up. Lowering the diaphragm is the hardest part of reverse breathing. It is very important now to practice the relaxing technique of smiling to the diaphragm and the abdomen.

(2) Exhale, releasing the pressure in the perineum and in the sexual organs. Exhale through the lower abdomen, allowing the pressure to protrude from the lower abdomen to all sides and not only the stomach. Relax, letting the fasciae expand while releasing and relaxing the chest totally. Smile down. Relax.

(3) Counting each inhalation and exhalation together as one, practice reverse breathing six, nine, and then eighteen times. Practice until you are able to control the diaphragm with your mind, commanding it to lower down or rise up.

2. The Pelvic and Urogenital Diaphragms

The body also contains a pelvic diaphragm and a urogenital diaphragm which are exceedingly important in transmitting energy in Iron Shirt. (Figure 2–5) The pelvic diaphragm is a muscular wall that extends across the lower part of the torso, suspended concavely downward from the level of the symphysis pubis (the joint of the pubic bones) in front and the sacrum (the back of the pelvis) in back. There are several organs that penetrate this muscular partition that lies between the pelvic cavity and the perineum. These are the urethra, the vagina and the rectum, and they are supported by the pelvic diaphragm. In fact, the pelvic diaphragm is the floor of the pelvic cavity which contains the large intestine, small intestine, bladder, kidneys, liver, spleen, and pancreas. It is the pelvic diaphragm that lifts up and maintains the shapes of the vital organs.

Below the pelvic diaphragm and above the perineum is another

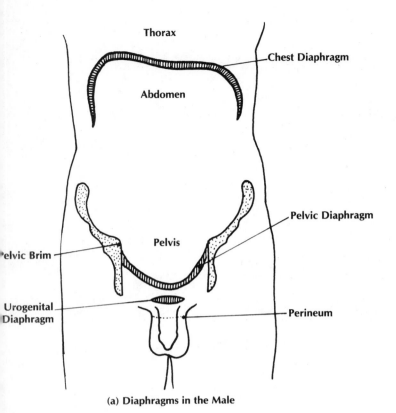

(a) Diaphrams in the Male

FIGURE 2-5

The pelvic and urogenital diaphrams are the major lower seals which prevent vital energy from leaking out the lower openings

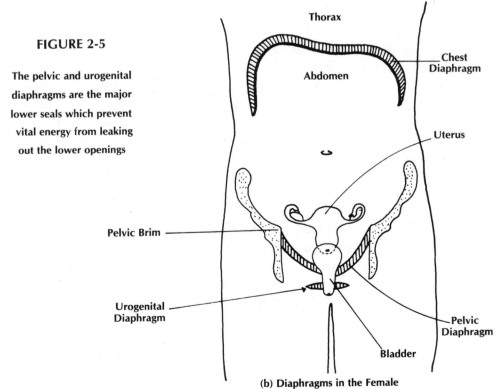

(b) Diaphrams in the Female

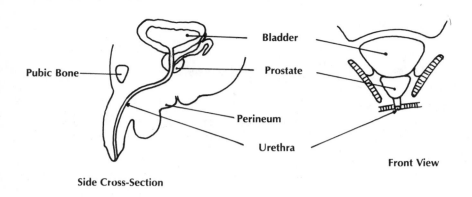

Bladder

Prostate

Pubic Bone

Perineum

Urethra

Side Cross-Section

Front View

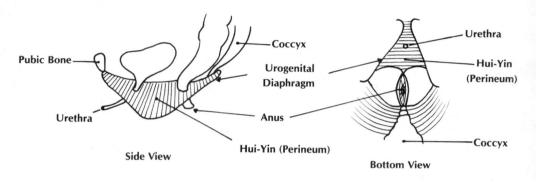

Pubic Bone

Coccyx

Urogenital
Diaphragm

Urethra

Anus

Hui-Yin (Perineum)

Side View

Urethra

Hui-Yin
(Perineum)

Coccyx

Bottom View

FIGURE 2-6

A closer view of the urogenital diaphragm in the male

muscular diaphragm called the urogenital diaphragm. (Figure 2–6)
This is penetrated by the urethra, while its underside is the attachment site of the root of the penis or vagina. The pudendal nerve connects the muscles of the urogenital diaphragm, the penis or vagina
and the anus. There is a membranous superficial fascia that attaches
to the back of this lowermost diaphragm that comes forward to engulf
the scrotum or vagina (which also contains muscle) and joins with
the abdominal wall. The importance of these anatomical structures
will become apparent as you progress in your work in Taoist Yoga,
especially in Iron Shirt I, II and III and in Taoist Secrets of Love (Seminal and Ovarian Kung Fu). These two diaphrams serve to assist the
flow of pressure to the vital organs and glands, and help tremendously to increase CHI pressure in the organs and the abdomen.
Knowing how to utilize and control these diaphragms will improve
your capabilities in all levels of the Healing Tao practice.

3. Iron Shirt Packing Process Breathing (CHI Pressure)

Packing Process Breathing is the most important breathing technique to master in the practice of Iron Shirt. It is used in all of the Iron Shirt postures and practicing it well will be a great aid in benefitting from the postures.

The Packing Process creates air pressure in a small space so that the body can have more pounds of pressure per square inch (psi). The importance of not only expanding the abdomen out in the front but allowing it to protrude on all sides has been stressed in the description of abdominal and reverse breathing. The same is true of Packing Breathing. The expansion of the front, back and sides occurs proportionately until the abdominal area becomes round like a ball. (Figure 2–7) Watch a child breathe and you will notice that his/her abdomen is round. In Chapter 1, we compared this phenomena to a tire which inflates to a certain number of pounds of air pressure (psi) in order to lift and support a car. By utilizing this process, the human body can store air pressure (energy) in various parts of the body. When the pressure (CHI) drops, all the organs will drop and stack on each other, dropping down and giving a greater burden to the pelvic and urogenital diaphragms. CHI pressure will help the organs hold their shape and uplift the organs into their own positions so that energy can flow easily. Thus, the CHI pressure serves as an energy charger of the organs.

The Taoists believe that the body has many openings: one front door, the sexual organ; one back door, the anus; and the seven open-

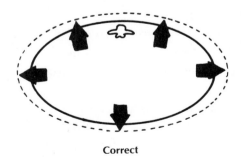

Correct

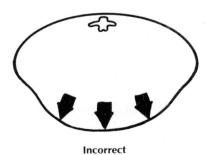

Incorrect

FIGURE 2-7

The abdomen during Packing Process Breathing becomes rounded like a ball

ings of its windows, two eyes, two ears, two nostrils, and one mouth. It is through these openings that energy can enter or leak from the body. In the practice of Iron Shirt, we learn to seal our bodies to prevent energy leakage and the loss of CHI pressure, enabling us to pack, condense and store energy in our bodies and organs. Pulling up the pelvic and urogenital diaphragms helps to seal the sexual organ and anus doors. Turning the attention of your senses down to the navel area will also help to seal the energy.

a. Preparation Using Abdominal and Reverse Breathing (Energizer Breathing)

Sit at the front edge of your chair (the best position for practicing the Microcosmic Orbit also). Place your tongue at the roof of your mouth to seal the leakage of tongue and heart energy. Listen inwardly to your kidneys and breathe inwardly to the lungs. Look inwardly to the liver, and all of the other organs as well, to seal the senses from the inside.

(1) Start with the first stage of Energizer Breathing; that is, abdominal breathing. (Figure 2–8(a)) Inhale slowly but strongly. Keep the chest relaxed and feel the area of the lower abdomen below the navel and perineum bulge. (Remember, abdominal and reverse breathing originates from the lower abdomen, approximately one and one-half inches below the navel.) Then, forcefully, exhale. Notice that when you exhale, the belly flattens toward the spine. (Figure 2–8(b)) Feel the sexual organs pull up. The perineal bulge diminishes. Learn to keep the stomach flat after exhaling. Inhale slowly again and allow the perineum to bulge as you do so. Repeat in multiples of eighteen to 36. The purpose is to energize the CHI and is also called "Fanning the Fire".

(2) When you are ready and feel that you have sunk the CHI downwards towards the navel, exhale so that the abdomen flattens towards the spine. The chest and sternum sink down, pressing and activating the thymus gland. Exhale once more and lower the diaphragm down. (Figure 2–8(c)) Hold for a while and then, using reverse abdominal breathing, inhale ten percent of your full capacity to the navel (ten percent means a short, little breath) while keeping the belly flat (Figure 2–8(d)), then relax the chest and belly. Try to keep the diaphragm low.

b. Building CHI Pressure

(3) Inhale about ten percent while contracting the pelvic and uro-genital diaphragms. (Figure 2–8(e)) Pull up the sexual organs and tighten the anus to seal in your energy. Compress the abdominal organs in three directions: above from the lowered diaphragm, below from the sexual organs, and in front from the abdominal wall. The

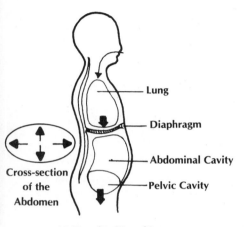

(a) Energizer Breathing

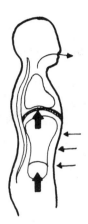

(b) Exhale. Flatten the
abdomen to the spine

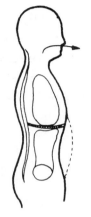

(c) Exhale and lower
the diaphragm

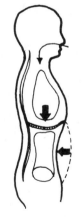

(d) Inhale ten percent,
keeping the belly flat

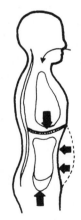

(e) Inhale ten percent,
contracting the pelvic
and urogenital diaphragms

FIGURE 2-8

Packing Process Breathing

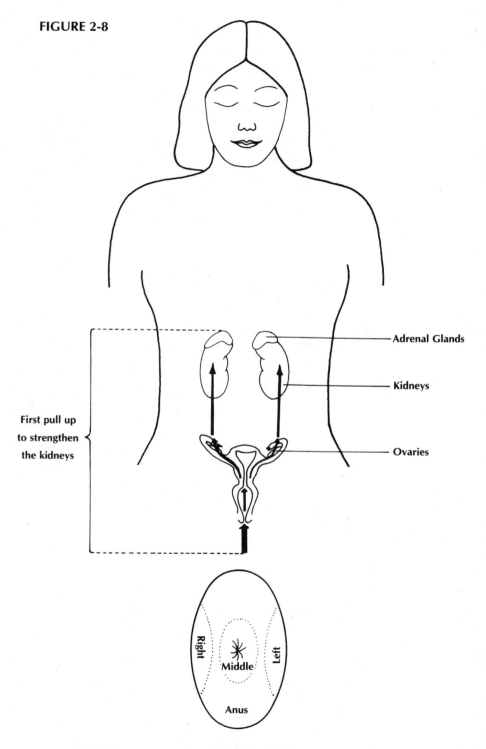

FIGURE 2-8

Adrenal Glands

Kidneys

Ovaries

First pull up
to strengthen
the kidneys

Right

Left

Middle

Anus

(f) Inhale ten percent. Contract the left and right anus. Bring CHI to the
left and right kidneys. Pack and wrap the kidneys

ribs and spine hold from behind. (Figure 2-2(b)) Inhale ten percent. Contract the left side of the anus, thereby bringing the CHI to the left kidney. Pack and wrap the energy around the left kidney and the adrenal glands. At the same time, pull in more of the left stomach towards the spine. Pull up the right anus and bring the CHI to the right kidney. At the same time, pull more on the right side of the abdomen wall, flattening it towards the spine. Pack and wrap the energy around the right and left kidneys. (Figure 2–8(f)) Hold this position for as long as you can.

Remember if the diaphragm becomes tight and pushed up, rub it with both hands to gently work the diaphragm so that it will drop down into a relaxed position. (Figure 2–4)

(4) When you can no longer hold your breath, inhale ten percent more air on top of the air that you already have inhaled. Contract the perineum more tightly, especially the sex organs. You can jerk a little, in order to pack the energy in the lower abdomen. Seal and limit the energy to a small area. You must maintain a relaxed chest and sink the sternum so that the diaphragm will stay soft and lowered. The stomach is flat and held in. Feel the pressure extend to the area of the sperm palace/ovary palace. (Figure 2–8(g)) Pull the sex organs and the anus up again and seal them so that no energy can leak out.

(5) Inhale ten percent more air. (You can exhale a little in order to inhale more air.) Contract the pelvic area and lower part of the abdomen, and hold this position for as long as possible. (Figure 2–8(h))

(6) Inhale ten percent more. Repeat. Feel the pressure build in the perineum. (Figure 2–8(i))

(7) By this time, it may seem that you cannot accommodate any more air, but if you exhale a little bit, bend forward slowly and direct your attention to the kidneys, feeling them expand on both sides and backwards, relaxing and trusting that the air will have room there, you will be able to inhale the last ten percent of your full capacity to that area in the back. (Figure 2–8(j)) Hold as long as possible. This will help to open the sides and back.

(8) Exhale. Sit up straight.

(9) Normalize breathing by using abdominal breathing.

When you exhale and relax at the end of such a session, you will

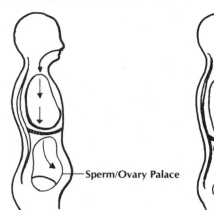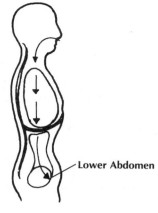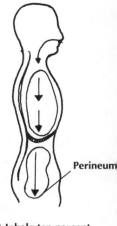

(g) Inhale ten percent
down to the
lower abdomen

—Sperm/Ovary Palace

(h) Inhale ten percent
down to the
pelvic area and
lower abdomen

—Lower Abdomen

(i) Inhale ten percent
down to the
perineum

Perineum

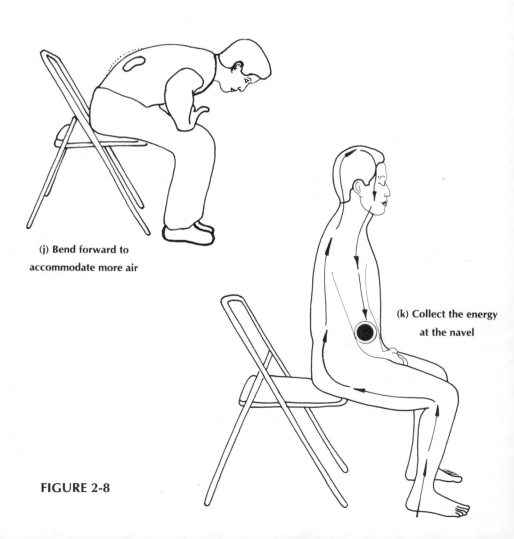

(j) Bend forward to
accommodate more air

(k) Collect the energy
at the navel

FIGURE 2-8

immediately experience heat or feel the energy run all around the body. Put the tongue to the palate. At this point you should meditate and circulate the Microcosmic Orbit for a few rounds. Collect the energy in the navel when you have finished. (Figure 2–8(k))

Using this breathing method, the organs are packed, compressed and strongly massaged. When you inhale, blood and energy (CHI) will rush in with great force to clear the organs out, making them progressively stronger and healthier.

If you feel energy stuck in the heart area, use both hands to brush the chest in a downward motion. In addition, you may want to do the Healing Sound for the heart (see the method described in the book, *Taoist Ways to Transform Stress into Vitality*) and walk around, shaking out the arms and legs.

4. Points To Remember in Practicing the Breathing Exercises

a. Always remember: DO NOT USE FORCE. Relax the chest so that the chest, sternum and diaphragm can sink down.

b. When packing, stay soft inside, not tense, at least for a good deal of the time. Soft energy is said to be unlimited.

c. Do no more than three cycles of packing per day for the first week. Gradually increase to six, nine and eighteen cycles per day. This exercise is much more strenuous than you might imagine. Energy, wrapped around the organs and pushed into the fasciae by opposing pressure, eventually increases the amount of energy stored in the fasciae and organs, protecting you against blows or unexpected injuries.

5. Preliminary Exercises

Here are some exercises which will be very helpful to you in the practice of Iron Shirt Chi Kung. All exercises should be performed as often as the body finds necessary, in multiples of three.

a. Check the Diaphragm

The following is a procedure to check that the diaphragm is lowered. First, press deeply on the stomach with the fingers of one hand directly below the sternum. You will feel a sharp pain that will tell you that you have pressed on the stomach. Next, inhale, allowing the abdomen to balloon out. Touch the diaphragm under the rib cage near the sternum, above the stomach. You will feel a pain which is quite different from stomach pains. Make sure you are relaxed so that the diaphragm lowers. *This is the most important part of Iron Shirt practice. Keep the diaphragm lowered at all times while using the packing process. This will prevent the CHI from congesting the lungs and heart and allow it to continue its course downward to the navel.*

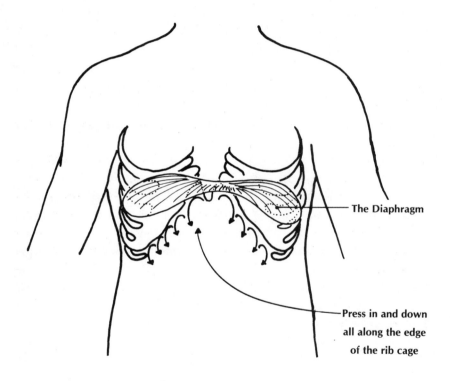

The Diaphragm

Press in and down all along the edge of the rib cage

FIGURE 2-9

Releasing Tension in the Diaphragm

b. Massage the Diaphragm

Many people have a very tight, stiff diaphragm which sticks to the rib cage. To release the diaphragm, you can massage above the rib cage: (a) massage along the rib cage from top to bottom; (b) use the index, third and fourth fingers to push downward from the rib cage, and feel the stretch of the diaphragm. (Figure 2–9) When the diaphragm is stretched, you will feel breathing to be easier and deeper. This can easily be accomplished in the morning when you rise.

c. Abdominal Breathing in a Lying Position

Your greatest reservoir of CHI is in the area of the navel. Concentrating on this area can increase CHI pressure and stimulate its flow. Your CHI always travels to where your attention and activity is centered. When you breathe high in the chest, your CHI goes there and, because CHI cannot be stored there, you will begin to feel distress. Abdominal breathing will avoid this problem.

This exercise will help you accomplish abdominal breathing in a lying position easily.

Lie flat on your back with the legs flat on the floor or with the feet on the floor and the knees raised just enough to allow the lower back to flatten against the floor. Place one hand on the sternum and the other hand on the lower abdomen. When you inhale, allow the belly to swell enough to raise the hand that you have resting on it, while the chest remains comparatively still. Do this to the count of nine, and then put the arms at the sides. Exhale. Breathe in for nine more such cycles. Breathe abdominally without using the hands. Then place the hands on the chest and lower the abdomen again and repeat the exercise. Be alert to this breathing process and not to how you feel. Put the hands at the sides of the body again, and realize what you have learned.

Repeat this exercise lying on one side and then the other. To give you stability in this position, bend the knees in front of you so that if someone were to look at you from above, you would look as if you were seated in a chair. When breathing, gradually feel the air expand from the lower lungs to the middle, the left, the right side and up, until the chest feels like a cylinder.

d. Abdominal Breathing on a Slant Board

This exercise will greatly increase the pressure and strength of the abdomen and strengthen the diaphragm.

Lie on a slant board with the head towards the floor while doing this same exercise. Using a weight on the lower abdomen while lying flat, breathe in so that the weight is raised as the diaphragm lowers. Exhale. The diaphragm goes back to its normal position and allows the belly to flatten and lower the weight. Practice this daily, increasing the weight once a week and you will soon acquire a great control in directing CHI to the lower abdomen while strengthening the abdominal muscles. By putting the board higher up on the wall, you can increase the demands made on the abdomen and diaphragm. This approach allows you to discover various ways of adapting to a new position and gain greater control. Always repeat in multiples of three to 36 times.

When you are proficient at abdominal breathing, you may go on to the next exercise.

e. Strengthening through Counter Pressure

For this exercise you will need a partner who will exert pressure on specific points of your body using a fist. Your partner should coordinate with you to determine the correct amount of pressure required for you to respond.

(1) Have your partner hold a fist against your solar plexus. (Figure 2–10) Inhale, directing your attention and your diaphragm to the point of contact, and produce a counter pressure. Practice this six times only, resting after each time, and you will see how quickly you have learned to respond.

(2) Your partner should hold a fist against your navel area. (Figure 2–11) Inhale, direct your attention and your diaphragm to the point of contact, and produce a counter pressure. Practice at this spot six times, resting after each time.

(3) Now, have your partner hold a fist against the lower abdominal area. Inhale and direct your attention and your diaphragm to this area, producing a counter pressure. Practice this exercise six times also, again resting after each time.

(4) Finally, ask your partner to hold a fist against each side separately, a little towards the back in the kidneys' areas (vulnerable areas which are easily hurt by a blow). (Figure 2–12) Inhale, direct your attention to the spot and produce a counter pressure. Do this six times,

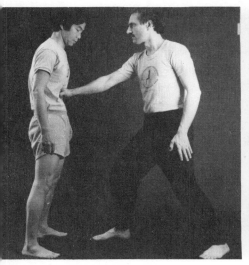

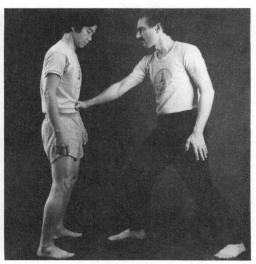

FIGURE 2-10

Your partner with his fist against your solar plexus

FIGURE 2-11

Your partner with his fist against your navel

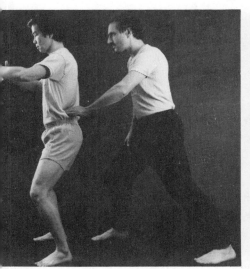

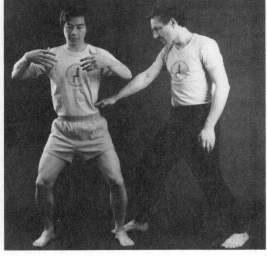

FIGURE 2-12

Your partner pressing with his fist against your side, towards the back, in
the kidney area

remembering to rest after each time. This exercise will begin to strengthen the kidneys' areas.

(5) Change places with your partner and repeat (1) through (4).

The effects of this simple exercise are widespread. It is invigorating, will mobilize an otherwise lax abdomen and can help you complete the Microcosmic Orbit quickly. If you cannot do it with a partner, use a wooden dowel affixed to a flat board. The dowel should be about one and one-half inches in diameter. Simply place the flat surface against a wall and lean against the dowel so that it presses against those places described above.

f. Abdominal Breathing in a Standing Position

Standing positions are mostly used in the Iron Shirt practice. It is harder to accomplish abdominal breathing in a standing position, thus you need to be more relaxed.

As your abdominal breathing in a lying position improves, you will more easily control it in a standing position. While standing, the fasciae have tension to hold the muscles and the organs. This exercise is to strenghthen the abdominal fasciae. This is a means of acquainting you with the way the mind and body work together and of learning how to bring energy to a fascial area. Stand with the feet a shoulders' width apart. Relax the entire body and make sure the diahpragm is lowered. Take a deep abdominal breath, swelling out the belly. Hold it as long as you can comfortably. Exhale. When you feel the need, inhale. Repeat this cycle in multiples of three.

g. Getting Energy to the Abdomen by Training the Mind to Direct It

After you have learned Iron Shirt Breathing, you can practice sending energy to the abdomen. With this exercise, you will gradually train your mind to direct and increase the CHI pressure at will to the upper, middle and lower abdominal areas, or to the left or right kidneys, packing, wrapping and energizing them, to the adrenal glands, the liver, the spleen, the pancreas, the lungs, the heart, the thymus gland, or the thyroid and parathyroid glands. (Figure 2–13) (In the advanced level, you will learn to direct CHI to other parts of the body as well.)

h. Practice—The Development of Iron Shirt Protection

Make your left hand into a fist, with the inside edge of the fist

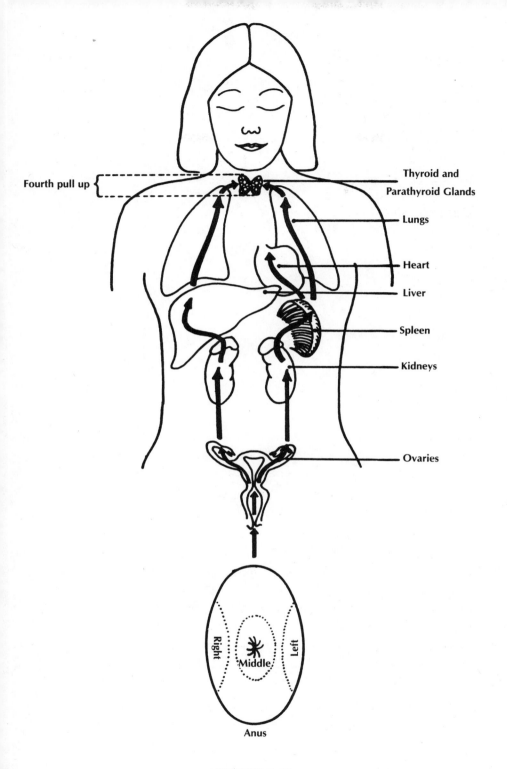

Fourth pull up

Thyroid and Parathyroid Glands

Lungs

Heart

Liver

Spleen

Kidneys

Ovaries

Right

Middle

Left

Anus

FIGURE 2-13

Train the mind to direct CHI to the organs and glands

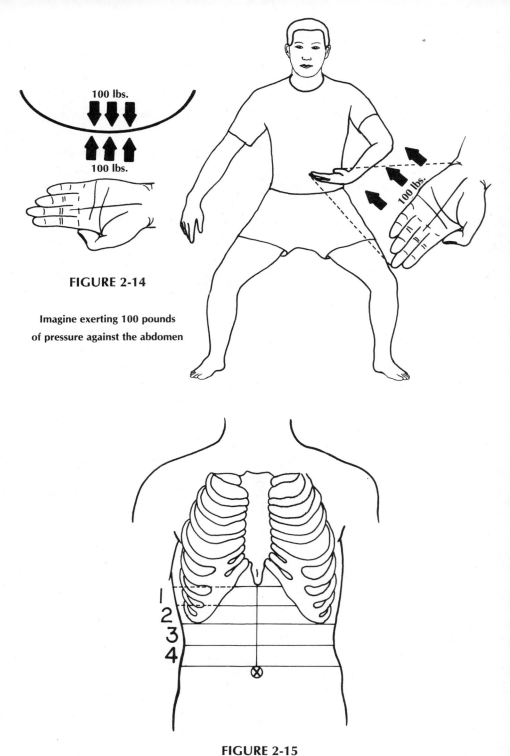

FIGURE 2-14

Imagine exerting 100 pounds
of pressure against the abdomen

100 lbs.

100 lbs.

100 lbs.

FIGURE 2-15

The Four Divisions of the Abdomen below the Sternum

facing inward as if it were holding a knife, and hold it over the abdominal area. Inhale. Imagine that CHI is filling the lower abdomen and that the edge of the fist is exerting 100 pounds of pressure against the abdomen. (Figure 2-14) Resist. Now relax. Inhale. Do not force the energy in any way. When you feel comfortable with this pressure, gradually increase it so that the body will be able to handle it. This prepares you so that if you were hit without any warning anywhere on the body, you could send CHI to those points to cushion the body and vital organs from harm.

Most people cannot take a punch to the stomach, which is located at the level of the solar plexus. With this training, you would be able to do just that. However, in the Taoist practice we do not encourage people to show off by taking a punch.

You must make sure you are relaxed throughout this exercise. Begin by "filling the abdomen with air". You can achieve this by concentrating on the area around and below the navel. The area from the navel to the sternum is divided into four parts. (Figure 2–15) Wherever you direct your attention, CHI appears and protects the area like an inflated rubber tire. Use no force at any time in this practice. Simply breathe into the area you want to cushion, and concentrate on it while gradually pushing your palm into it. Do this systematically so that you cover all the body surfaces that you can reach.

Once you develop energy in the region between the sternum and the navel sufficient to protect you against unexpected injury, the rest of the abdomen is more easily protected. The counterpressure that is created drives CHI into the fasciae. When the deep fasciae fill with CHI pressure, the CHI pressure will spread out to the second layer of the fasciae. (For more detailed information regarding fasciae, see Chapter 4.) Soon, as you increase pressure in the abdomen, you will be able to move the CHI pressure around the abdominal area. Practice this constantly in conjunction with all of the Iron Shirt exercises.

Once you have become proficient with the hand, you can use a short stick. Press the stick in the abdominal area and push in as you bring the CHI pressure to the area to counteract the stick.

B. Summary of Iron Shirt Breathing

The breathing processes explained in this Chapter may seem to be numerous but, in fact, all relate and lead to Iron Shirt breathing.

1. Exercises to Improve Abdominal Breathing

a. Abdominal Breathing in a Lying Position

(1) Lie supine, legs flexed or extended, hands on belly. Inhale nine counts. Raise hands. Exhale. Repeat nine times with your hands at your sides.

(2) Lie supine, legs flexed or extended, hands on chest and lower abdomen. Inhale nine counts, allowing the belly to rise. Exhale. Repeat nine times with your hands at your sides.

(3) Repeat (1) and (2) on each side with knees flexed.

b. Abdominal Breathing on a Slant Board

(1) On a slant board, using a weight on the belly, inhale, raising the weight. Hold. Exhale.

(2) Lower the weight. Repeat, adding to the weight on a weekly basis. Repeat in multiples of three, nine, eighteen and 36.

c. Strengthening Through Counter Pressure

Use mind and body to direct pressure from within against an outside force, concentrating CHI in a particular area of fascia.

d. Abdominal Breathing in a Standing Position

(1) Stand with feet a shoulders' width apart. Inhale and hold as long as comfortable. Exhale. Repeat in multiples of three.

2. Iron Shirt Chi Kung Packing Process Breathing

a. Abdominal Breathing

Begin with abdominal breathing, expanding the lower abdomen.

b. Lower the Diaphragm

Lower the diaphragm upon inhalation while keeping the chest relaxed. Exhale, flattening the stomach, and feel the pull of the pelvic and urogenital diaphragms and sexual organs.

c. Reverse Abdominal Breathing

When you have brought the energy down to the navel, begin reverse breathing with an exhalation, flattening down the stomach. When inhaling, relax the chest and maintain a flattened stomach.

d. Slightly Contract the Pelvic and Urogenital Diaphragm

Contract the pelvic and urogenital diaphragm and, at the same time, slightly pull up the anus, and pull up the testicles or contract the vagina.

e. Packing Process Breathing

Begin Packing Process Breathing with an inhalation. Using the packing process, seal and limit the energy to a small area. The diaphragm is lowered. The stomach is flattened and held in. Pull up the sexual organs and anus and seal them so that no energy can leak out of these three areas.

f. Pack the Organs with CHI

The energy goes back, filling out and packing the kidneys' areas.

g. Exhale and Relax

Exhale and let the CHI out. Relax.

C. The Cranial, Respiratory and Sacral Pump Functions

Contained and protected within your spinal column and skull is the very "heart" of your nervous system. Cushioning it is the cerebrospinal fluid, cerebro for the head and spinal for the vertebrae. This fluid, as described by the Taoists in ancient times, is circulated by two pumps. One is in the sacrum and is known as the sacral pump. The other is in the region of your upper neck and head and is known as the cranial pump. Many people who have been able to feel these pumps working have reported feeling a "big bubble" of energy travel up their spine during Packing Breathing.

1. Sacral Pump (Figure 2–16)

The sacrum consists of five pieces of bone when we are young;

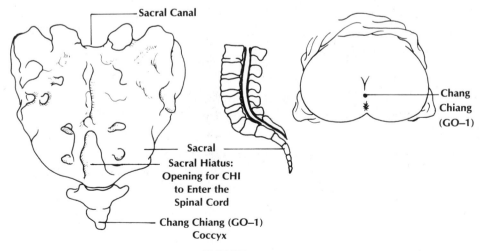

FIGURE 2-16

when we grow up these five bones fuse into one piece. Taoists regard the sacrum as a pump which will help to hold the sexual energy coming from the sperm/ovaries and perineum and transform the energy, at the same time giving it an upward thrust. It is similar to a way station, refining the sperm/ovaries' energy as it circulates in the body. In the Iron Shirt practice we tilt the sacrum to the back, or against a wall, exerting force to straighten the sacrum. This helps to activate the sacral pump to pump the spinal cord fluid up.

2. Cranial Pump

The cranium of the skull has long been regarded by Taoists as a major pump for the circulation of energy from the lower centers to the higher centers. Medical research has recently confirmed that minute movements of the joints of the eight cranial bones occur during breathing. (Figure 2–17) Cranial movement is responsible for the production and function of the cerebrospinal fluid surrounding the brain and spinal cord, which fluid is necessary for normal brain, nerve and energy patterns in the entire body.

Improper cranial respiratory function develops for many reasons. It may have been present from birth. At this time the skull is soft and moveable and the trip down the birth canal could jam a baby's skull, or it may be the result of a difficult birth in which forceps were used. It may also occur later in life. A bump on the head coming from a certain direction while the person is breathing in the specific manner that allows the bone to move can cause improper cranial respiratory function. Auto accidents causing whiplash very often are the cause of cranial faults. Since cranial faults affect the flow of the fluid and the brain, nerve and energy patterns of the entire body, symptoms can develop anyplace. Strengthening the cranial joints can increase energy and alleviate symptoms, such as headaches, sinus problems, visual disturbances and neck problems.

In Taoism, cultivation of the movement of the pelvis, perineum, urogenital diaphragm, anus, and the sacrum and cranial pumps are very important in helping to move the life-force and sexual energy up to the higher center. The Iron Shirt Chi Kung Packing Process activates these pumps using various methods, e.g. mind control, muscle action,

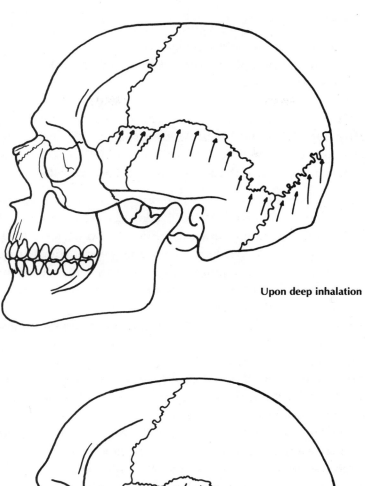

Upon deep inhalation

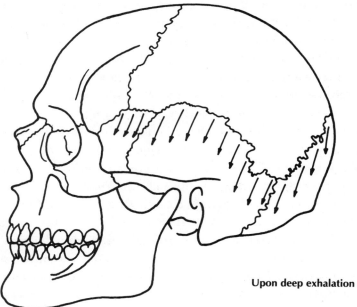

Upon deep exhalation

FIGURE 2-17

Micromovement of Cranial Bones

clenching of the teeth and tightening of the neck, and pressing the tongue to the palate. All of these methods will help to activate the eight pieces of cranial bone.

D. The Microcosmic Orbit Meditation

1. Circulate Your CHI in the Microcosmic Orbit (Figure 2–18)

In the preceding breathing exercises, you have been asked at certain points to circulate the Microcosmic Orbit. Your life-force energy thus must be circulated through specific pathways in the body efficiently and safely to be used for healing and growth. The Microcosmic Orbit circulation uses the power of the mind to help activate the sacral and cranial pumps into pumping the life-force energy throughout the body.

It is much easier to cultivate your energy if you first understand the major paths of energy circulation in the body. The nervous system in humans is very complex and is capable of directing energy wherever it is needed. The ancient Taoist Masters discovered that there are many channels of energy flow. However, two energy channels carry an especially strong current.

One channel is called the "Functional" or "Yin" Channel. It begins at the perineum, the point located at the base of the trunk, midway between the testicles/vagina and the anus. It goes up the front of the body past the sex organ, stomach, organs, heart, and throat and ends at the tip of the tongue. The second channel, called the "Governor" or "Yang" channel, also starts at the perineum but goes up the back of the body. It flows from the perineum upwards into the tailbone and the sacral pump and then up through the spine into the brain and the cranial pump, finally flowing back down to the roof of the mouth.

The tongue is like a switch that connects these two currents— when it is touched to the roof of the mouth just behind the front teeth, the energy can flow in a circle up the spine and back down the front. The two channels form a single circuit that energy loops around. This vital current of energy circulates past the major organs and nervous systems of the body in a loop, giving cells the juice created from organ energy and smiling energy that is necessary to grow, heal, and func-

The Functional Channel **The Governing Channel**

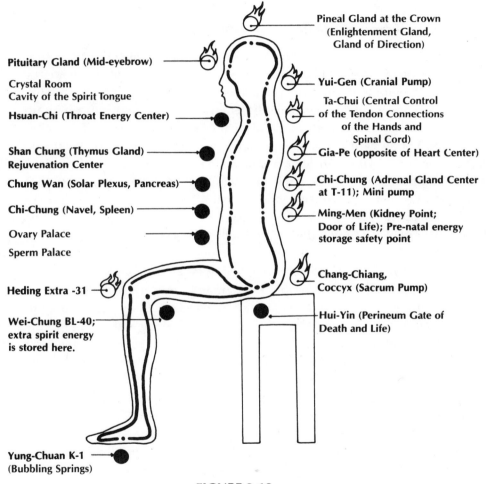

Pituitary Gland (Mid-eyebrow)

Crystal Room
Cavity of the Spirit Tongue

Hsuan-Chi (Throat Energy Center)

Shan Chung (Thymus Gland)
Rejuvenation Center

Chung Wan (Solar Plexus, Pancreas)

Chi-Chung (Navel, Spleen)

Ovary Palace

Sperm Palace

Heding Extra -31

Wei-Chung BL-40;
extra spirit energy
is stored here.

Yung-Chuan K-1
(Bubbling Springs)

Pineal Gland at the Crown
(Enlightenment Gland,
Gland of Direction)

Yui-Gen (Cranial Pump)

Ta-Chui (Central Control
of the Tendon Connections
of the Hands and
Spinal Cord)

Gia-Pe (opposite of Heart Center)

Chi-Chung (Adrenal Gland Center
at T-11); Mini pump

Ming-Men (Kidney Point;
Door of Life); Pre-natal energy
storage safety point

Chang-Chiang,
Coccyx (Sacrum Pump)

Hui-Yin (Perineum Gate of
Death and Life)

FIGURE 2-18

Learn to circulate your CHI in the Microcosmic Orbit. The tongue touches the
roof of the palate to complete the circuit of the Governing and Functional Channels

tion, and spreading vitality throughout the body. This circulating energy is the Microcosmic Orbit, and forms the basis of acupuncture. Western medical research has already acknowledged acupuncture as being clinically effective, although scientists admit they cannot explain why the system works. The Taoists, on the other hand, have been studying the subtle energy points in the body for thousands of years and have verified in detail the importance of each channel.

2. The Importance of the Microcosmic Orbit

By opening up this Microcosmic Orbit and keeping it clear of physical or mental blockages, it is possible to pump the life-force energy up the spine. If this channel is blocked by tension, then learning to circulate the Microcosmic Orbit is an important step to opening up the blocks in the body to circulate and revitalize all parts of the mind and body. Otherwise, when intense pressure builds in the head, taking such forms as headaches, hallucinations, and insomnia, much of the life-force energy escapes through the eyes, ears, nose and mouth and is lost. This is like trying to heat a room while all the windows are open.

The way to open the Microcosmic Orbit is by sitting in meditation for a few minutes each morning as you practice the Inner Smile. An essential Taoist technique described in detail in *Taoist Ways to Transform Stress into Vitality,* the Inner Smile is a means of connecting visual relaxation and the ability to concentrate. Allow your energy to complete the loop by letting your mind flow along with it. Start in the eyes, and mentally circulate with the energy as it goes down the front through your tongue, throat, chest and navel and then up the tailbone and spine to the head.

At first it may feel as though nothing is happening, but eventually the current will begin to feel warm in some places as it loops around. The key is simply to relax and try to bring your mind directly into the part of the loop being focused on. This is different from visualizing an image inside your head of what that part of the body looks like or is feeling. Do not use your mind as if it were a television picture. Experience the actual CHI flow. Relax and let your mind flow with the CHI in the physical body along a natural circuit to any desired point, e.g. the navel, perineum, etc.

Study of the Microcosmic Orbit is recommended to all students who truly seek to master the techniques of Iron Shirt. Progress to the higher levels of transforming CHI and our creative energy to spiritual energy, without first learning the Microcosmic Orbit, is very difficult. Some people may already be "open" in these channels or relaxed when they are close to nature. The benefits of the Microcosmic Orbit extend beyond facilitating the flow of life-force energy and include prevention of aging and the healing of many illnesses, ranging from high blood pressure, insomnia and headaches to arthritis.

E. Perineum Power

In Iron Shirt practice, we will utilize "Perineum Power" to direct CHI to the areas, organs and glands that you wish to energize in order to pack and increase the CHI in that region. "Perineum Power" will be used in all Iron Shirt positions.

1. The Anus is Connected to Organ Energy

The perineum (Hui-yin) region includes the anus and sexual organs. The various sections of the anus region are closely linked with the organs' CHI. The Chinese term Hui-yin (perineum) means the collection point of all the Yin energy, or the lowest abdominal energy collection point. It is also known as the Gate of Death and Life. This point lies between the two main gates. One, called the front gate, is the sexual organ which is the big life-force opening. Here the life-force energy can easily leak out and deplete the organ's function. The second gate, or back gate, is the anus. This gate can also easily lose life-force when not sealed or closed tightly through muscular toning. In the Tao practices, especially in the Tao Secrets of Love and Iron Shirt, the perineum's power to tighten, close and draw the life-force back up the spine is an important practice. Otherwise, our life-force and sexual energy can become a "river of no return."

2. The Anus Region is Divided into Five Parts

The anus is divided into five regions: (a) middle, (b) front, (c) back, (d) left, and (e) right. (Figure 2–19)

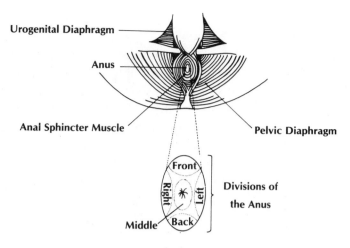

FIGURE 2-19

The anus is divided into five regions

a. The Middle Part

The middle of the anus CHI is connected with the organs as follows: the vagina-uterus, the aorta and vena cava, stomach, heart, thyroid and parathyroids, pituitary gland, pineal and top of the head. (Figure 2–20)

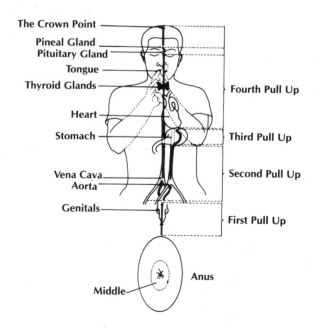

FIGURE 2-20

The Middle Part

b. The Front Part

The front of the anus CHI is connected with the following organs: the prostate gland, bladder, small intestine, stomach, thymus gland, and front part of the brain. (Figure 2–21(a) and (b))

(a) The Front Part in the Male

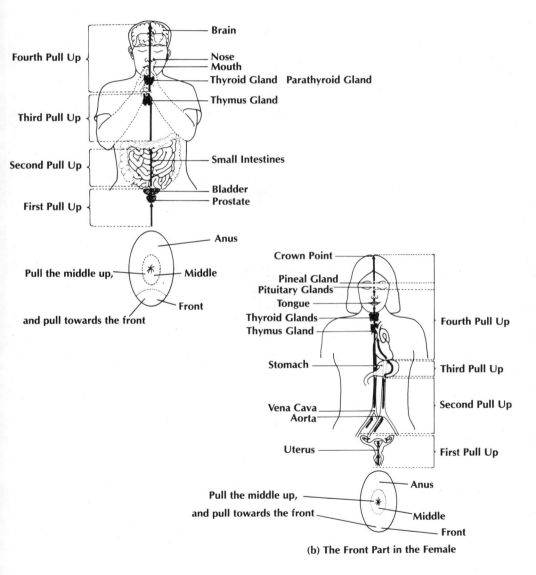

(b) The Front Part in the Female

FIGURE 2-21

c. The Back Part

The back part of the anus CHI is connected with the organ energies of: the sacrum, lower lumbars, twelve thoracic vertebrae, seven cervical vertebrae, and small brain (cerebellum). (Figure 2–22)

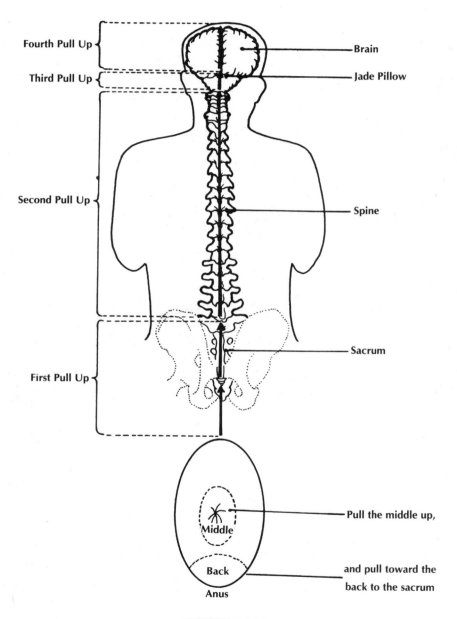

FIGURE 2-22

The Back Part

d. The Left Part

The left part of the anus CHI is connected with the organ energies of: the left ovary, the large intestine, left kidney, left adrenal gland, spleen, left lung and left hemisphere of the brain. (Figure 2–23 (a) and (b))

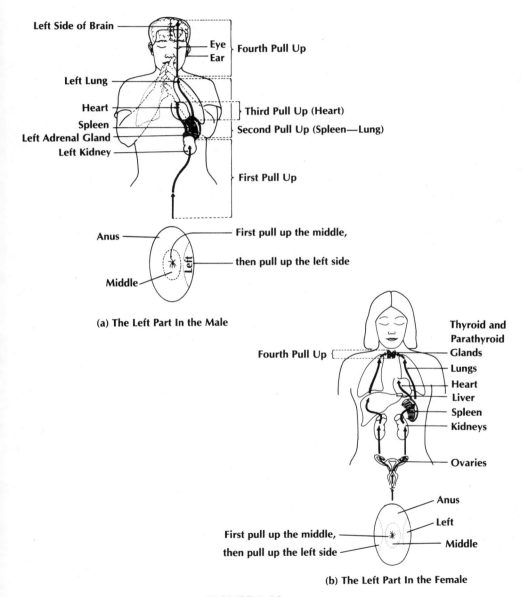

(a) The Left Part In the Male

(b) The Left Part In the Female

FIGURE 2-23

The Left Part

e. The Right Part

The right part of the anus CHI is connected with the organ energies as follows: the right ovary, the large intestine, right kidney, adrenal gland, liver, gall bladder, right lung and right hemisphere of the brain. (Figure 2-24 (a) and (b)).

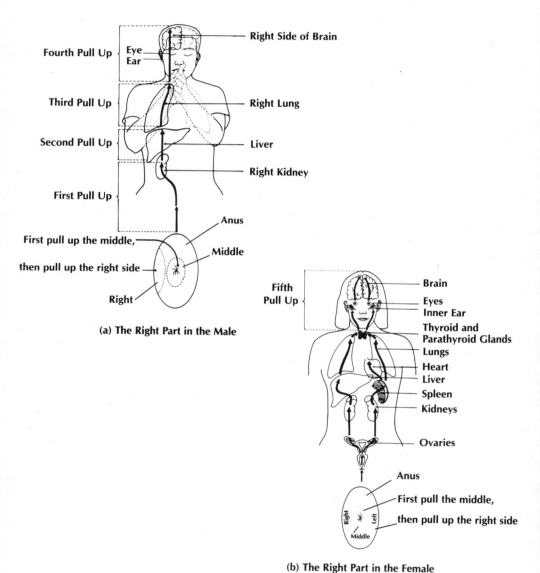

(a) The Right Part in the Male

(b) The Right Part in the Female

FIGURE 2-24

76   **The Right Part**

FIGURE 2-25

Wrap the organs, encircling them with CHI energy

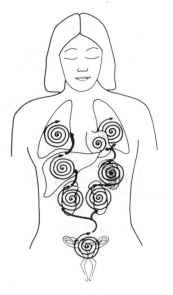

By contracting the anus in different parts you can bring more CHI to the organs and glands, and the effects of the massage will increase. (Figure 2-25)

F. Precautions

The following is a warning to practitioners with high blood pressure, emotional instability, heart or chest pain, or any acute illness.

1. If you have high blood pressure, check with a doctor before attempting the practice of Iron Shirt. Do not do the exercises and breathing techniques strenuously.

2. Women should not do Iron Shirt breathing during a menstrual cycle, but may practice the structure, standing CHI meditation and Bone Breathing. If pregnant, do not practice Iron Shirt Packing Breathing; use only energizer breathing and standing CHI meditation.

3. Be sure that the diaphragm is lowered while practicing these exercises to avoid accumulating energy in the heart and to facilitate the flow of the Microcosmic Orbit.

4. After practicing the postures, while bringing the energy down, be sure to place the tongue on the roof of the mouth to collect all energy from the head (the Governor Channel). Take the energy down from the head, slow it down in the solar plexus, and then store it in the navel.

3. PRACTICE OF POSTURES

There is an integral relationship between strong, unblocked CHI flow and good structural alignment. Proper practice of Iron Shirt, as well as all other Taoist exercises, will lead to a dramatic improvement in structural health, as well as increased CHI flow. A refined understanding of the structural interrelationships of the body is inherent in Iron Shirt.

Because of poor postural habits, many people have developed serious structural distortions and have no natural sense of the body in appropriate alignment. If these distortions are carried over into Iron Shirt practice, much effectiveness is lost and bad habits perpetuated. In effect, one is practicing the very problems that need to be corrected.

I. DEVELOPING THE IRON SHIRT HORSE STANCE USING A WALL

The following exercise demonstrates how to use a wall to align yourself perfectly in the Iron Shirt Horse Stance used in Embracing the Tree, Holding the Golden Pot and the Phoenix postures. These postures will be described fully in this chapter.

This wall position is a variation of the Structural Training Position against a Wall which is described in Chapter 4. As your practice continues, you will develop the feeling of proper alignment and will be able to follow the same principles without a wall. Whenever you practice your alignment against the wall, when you feel you can hold the position, step away from it and apply the same principles. After you have learned to adopt the correct stance without the wall, occasionally practice against it again to check yourself. Once you are skilled, occasional use of the wall will allow you greatly to increase your spinal lengthening when you practice.

Use this wall position to practice alignment by itself as well as with the breathing used in Embracing the Tree and the other excersises in which packing is done. Practicing the full exercise with Packing Breathing while against the wall will help to insure that you can maintain the alignment while in the much more dynamic state of packing and energy circulation.

At first, applying some of these details may seem difficult or unclear. However, as your body opens up, you will gradually be able to apply each detail easily and naturally. Since these principles represent application of the basic design characterisics of your body structure, you will feel more and more as you practice that your body will naturally fit into these "grooves".

A. Sequence of Practice in Using a Wall to Develop the Iron Shirt Horse Stance (Figure 3–1)

1. Distance Between Feet

Stand with the left foot a few inches away from the wall. The foot should be straight along the second toe, or just slightly turned out at the heel. To measure the proper distance between the feet, touch the knee of the right leg to the heel of the left foot. Place the ball of the right big toe in line with the ball of the left big toe so that both are

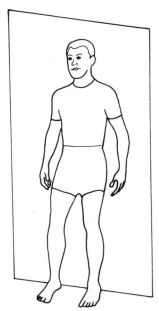

FIGURE 3-1

Horse Stance Using a Wall

the same distance away from the wall. Now, as you stand up, rotate the right foot around the ball of the big toe. Both heels will then be the same distance from the wall, and the feet will be the correct distance apart.

2. Foot Alignment

First, feel that you firmly contact the ground with the balls of the big toes. Then, spread the toes by widening the feet across the balls. Now equalize the weight over the whole foot by equalizing the weight on the following three points: the ball of the large toe, the ball of the last two toes, and the middle of the heel. (Figure 3–2) The toes should remain relaxed and not be grasping the floor. Remember that the feet are the foundation of your stance. As these details become natural, your practice will be much stronger, and you will experience greater body-mind integration. Proper foot alignment is the basis of understanding.

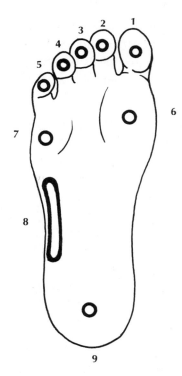

FIGURE 3-2

The Nine Points of the Foot

3. Distance from the Wall

The feet should be the right distance from the wall so that with the spine flattened to the wall, you do not feel like you are leaning back. If the wall were suddenly removed, you would not need to adjust yourself to keep from falling back.

4. Rooting with the Feet

When practicing those parts of Embracing the Tree and Rooting that call for strongly grasping the ground with the toes, feel that this clawing begins at the balls of the feet, not at the toes themselves. Accentuate this grasping at the big toe in particular and there will be much stronger rooting because the foot is used in a more complete and integrated fashion.

5. Knees

Bend the knees so that the kneecaps are directly over the toes. Bend the knees no farther than the ends of the big toes. The knees can be bent less than this, but eventually should be bent this far to insure maximum development of strength.

6. Pelvis

First, allow the lower spine to flatten firmly against the wall for as long as this can be done without discomfort. Then, place your hands on the tops of the thighs at the crease where the thighs connect to the pelvis. With the lower spine flattened to the wall, you will feel that the tendon in the front of the thigh and slightly to the inside is very tight. Now, rotate the pelvis slightly so that the lower spine comes away from the wall. You will feel this tendon relax. You should barely be able to place a flat hand between your lower spine and the wall. This will also increase the crease at the junction of the thigh and pelvis. Continue to feel that the sacrum is stretching the spine down.

7. Pelvic Tilt

As your practice of Iron Shirt continues and your attention is focused to the sacral area, the pelvic tilt is used. This is accomplished by strongly pushing against the wall at the sacral area while maintaining the other structural details. As you strongly push back to the wall, your spine will arch slightly more, and you will feel the muscles around the sacrum become very firm. As this happens, it is very important to feel that you are also stretching the sacrum further down the wall. (Figure 3–3) If you are doing this properly, you will feel a strong force around the sacrum with only a small added arch in the lower spine.

8. Middle Back

To insure that this pelvic aligning does not arch the middle spine, maintain the pelvic tilt position, and push back gently, but firmly, the back lower ribs, simultaneously lifting them slightly higher up the

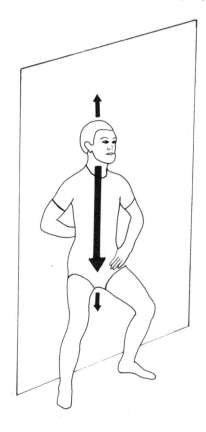

FIGURE 3-3

The Pelvic Tilt

wall. During this procedure you will feel the middle and lower back lengthen. (Figure 3–3) This is the work of the psoas muscles.

9. Head/Neck/UpperBack

Remain in the pelvic tilt position and bring as much of the upper spine as flat to the wall as possible without strain. Maintain the head as if it is being gently pushed back from the upper lip and simultaneosly lifted by its crown. (Figure 3–3) Again, for many people the head held in this way will not touch the wall. This is usually because of excessive curvature of the upper spine, which can be eliminated by practice of the Iron Bridge, the Backbend and Door Hanging. (The Iron Bridge is described subsequently in this chapter; see Chapter 4 for descriptions of the Backbend and Door Hanging.)

10. T–11 Thrust

When CHI energy is brought to the adrenal energy center (the T–11 point, located at the top of the kidneys at the point of the adrenal gland, or at the bottom edge of the rib cage at the spine) and packed in the kidney area, it is necessary to lean forward and thrust the T–11 area back. To feel this on the wall, simply keep the T–11 area firmly pressed against the wall and round the rest of the spine above this point away from the wall, while maintaining the other alignment principles. By practicing against the wall in this way, it is possible to feel this thrust very strongly, as when practicing with a partner pushing at that point.

11. Shoulders

Place the arms in any one of the arm positions as described in the first four Iron Shirt exercises in this chapter. Then move the shoulder blades firmly back to the wall so that the whole area of each shoulder blade is in firm contact with the wall. Now round the shoulders forward, feeling the shoulder blades move away from the wall, until just the spine and, if possible, the area between the inner edges of the shoulder blades remain on the wall.

12. Head/Neck (C–7, the Base of the Neck, and C–1, the Base of the Skull)

After rounding the shoulders forward, push back gently, but firmly, at C–7, the bone at the base of the neck, and at C–1, the bone at the base of the skull. The chin will tuck in as you do this. When bringing the CHI to these two points, you will drop the chin, bringing it closer to the chest. Even when pushing strongly, neither point will touch the wall. Until that point in the excercise is reached, however, push back less strongly (particularly at C–7) to insure that alignment with the upper spine and neck remains correct. (Figure 3–4) If done properly, pushing back at C–7 after rounding the shoulders forward will increase the rounding of the shoulders, and you will feel that the shoulders have become "locked" in place.

13. "Locking" the Structure

Lock the knees and do not move them. As you concentrate on the knees, they will feel as though they are simultaneously being pushed in and out. Then push the knees outward. You will feel a spiraling effect from the knees to the ground as if your legs were screws being screwed down into the earth. In Embracing the Tree, similarly lock the arms, but do not move them. Feel that the elbows are simultaneously being pushed in and pulled out as if the arms were screws being moved by the spiraling action of the forearm. You can also feel this locking action of the elbows and the knees if you imagine that you are straightening the joint, but without actually doing so. Locking these joints greatly improves strength, stability and CHI flow. Practice the Wall Stance and the Embracing the Tree posture for a while, until you can feel you are able to hold the position.

B. Summary of Practice For Using a Wall to Develop Iron Shirt Horse Stance Basic Alignment

1. Feet: Measure the proper distance of the feet from each other and from the wall. Align each foot.

2. Lower Back: Lean against the wall with the lower spine flat, if possible.

3. Head/Neck/UpperBack: Bring as much of the upper spine as pos-

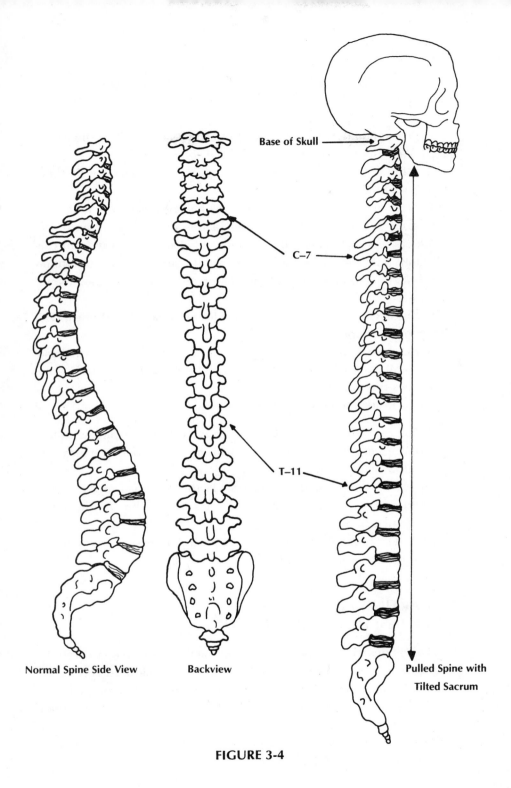

Base of Skull

C–7

T–11

Normal Spine Side View

Backview

Pulled Spine with
Tilted Sacrum

FIGURE 3-4

sible flat to the wall, with the head held as if it is pushed back from the upper lip and lifted by its crown. The back of the head may or may not touch the wall.

4. Pelvis: Rotate the pelvis back until the thigh tendon is more relaxed. Feel that the sacrum is pulling the spine down.

5. Middle Back: Bring the lower ribs firmly to the back wall, then stretch them up slightly higher on the wall.

6. Arms/Shoulders: Position the arms for one of the first four Iron Shirt exercises. Flatten the shoulder blades to the wall. Round the shoulders forward, feeling the shoulder blades move away from the wall until only the spine and, if possible, the area between the inner edges of the shoulder blades remains on the wall. Lock the elbows and knees.

7. Chest: Check that the chest muscles are relaxed. The chest will be somewhat depressed.

8. Head/Neck: Gently, but firmly, push back at C–7 and at the base of the skull. Extend up from the crown of the head. The back of the head does not touch the wall.

Special Alignment During the Exercises:

9. Rooting with the Feet: "Claw" with the feet by grasping with the balls of the feet first, particularly the balls of the big toes. The toes will then follow in grasping the ground.

10. Pelvic Tilt: Rotate the pelvis back farther as you strongly extend the sacrum down the wall. Feel the muscles around the sacrum firmly push against the wall.

11. T–11 Thrust: Push the T–11 area firmly to the wall as you bring the rest of the upper spine away from the wall.

II. STARTING POSITION FOR ALL EXERCISES: EMBRACING THE TREE

We will describe the positions of Embracing the Tree very carefully in a detailed, step-by-step explanation in Part A below. In Part B, we will give a sequence of practice, which will give you a complete sequential picture to follow without distraction. Practice as you read Part A first. Then, join all the steps together by following Part B. Part C is a summary of the sequence of practice. Utilize the Horse Stance with the assistance of the wall to improve your structure.

A. Embracing the Tree (Explanation of Procedure)

Embracing the Tree is the Master Stance practice. This practice joins many body structures and tendons (CHI channels) together into one system. In the beginning it seems difficult, quite like putting a puzzle together. However, if you begin this practice by taking one step at a time, practicing each one until you can master it, then moving on to the next step, you will find this practice much easier to do. Once you have mastered the Horse Stance on the wall, you will find it much easier to practice Embracing the Tree.

1. The Correct Stance

The correct distance between the feet in all Iron Shirt stances is the length of the lower leg from knee to toes. (Figure 3–5(a)) Beginners may wish to place feet slightly farther apart, but the standard position yields the quickest results. (Figure 3–5(b),(c) and (d))

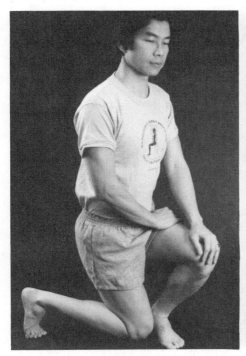
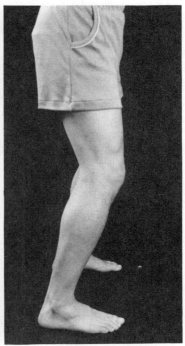

(a) Finding the Standard Position of the Feet   **(b) Rooting the Feet**

FIGURE 3-5

Embracing the Tree—Rooting

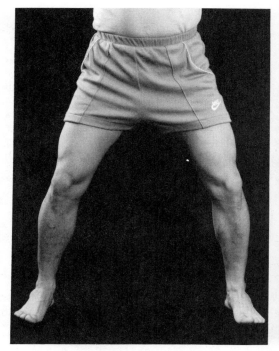 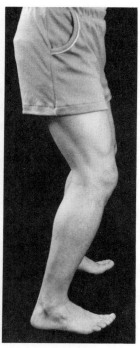

(c) Incorrect Rooting—Front View

(d) Incorrect Rooting
—Side View

FIGURE 3-5

2. Rooting of the Feet

As previously discussed, rooting is a very important practice in the
Tao System which begins with the physical practice and builds into
the higher, or spiritual, practice. Like the foundation of a building, the
Rooting Practice makes a strong foundation upon which to build,
making the structure last longer.

To root is to surrender yourself to the pull of gravity while maintaining a structural skeletal alignment which supports the body in an
upright posture.

In beginning the physical part of rooting, the soles of the feet (K–
1) are the places where Mother Earth's healing energy enters. When
the soles are open, you can feel the soles "sucking" and having a connection with the ground. This healing energy passes into the body
through the soles and will nourish the organs and the glands.

Like the roots of a tree, the feet support the entire structure. (Figure 3–6) It is important to distribute your weight solidly and evenly

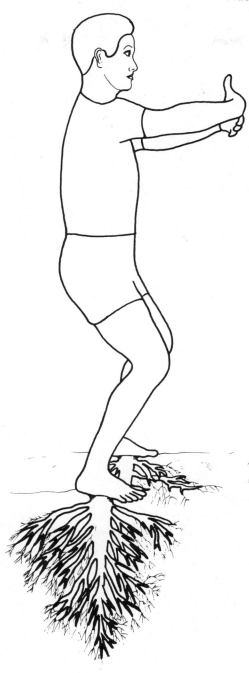

FIGURE 3-6

Feeling Rooted to the Earth

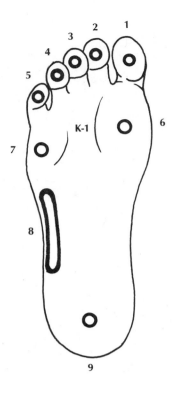

FIGURE 3-7

K–1 and the Nine Points of the Foot

on the whole foot. We divide the foot into nine parts, or nine bases: (1)big toe, (2)second toe, (3)third toe, (4)fourth toe, (5)small toe, (6)big ball, (7)small ball, (8)outer edge, and (9)heel. (Figure 3–7)

You must feel that the nine parts are evenly contacting the ground. Feel and check which parts are too tense or have too much pressure on them. This can cause the body to misalign and the spine to tilt to one side. Over a long period of time, improper alignment can cause spinal cord or disc problems.

The big toe joins with the tendons of the thumb (Figure 3–8), and the little toe joins with the tendons of the pinky finger (Figure 3–9); thus, all the tendons of the body are connected, increasing your rooting power. Slightly moving the feet inward, thereby pointing the toes in, will help to make the connection of the big toes and the thumb. In this posture, imagine you have roots extending down into the ground.

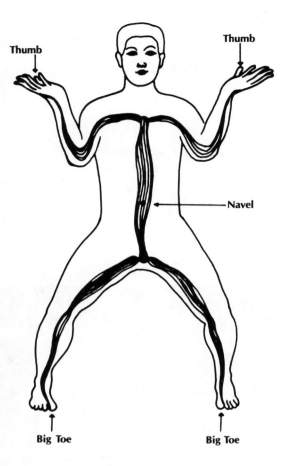

Thumb

Thumb

Navel

Big Toe

Big Toe

FIGURE 3-9

The tendons of the
big toes join with the
tendons of the thumbs

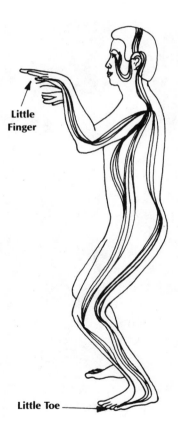

Little
Finger

Little Toe

FIGURE 3-8

The tendons of the
little toes join with the
tendons of the little finger

Note that if, at this point, the toes and ball of the foot were raised, the practitioner could easily be pushed over.

In the spiritual level of rooting, it is important to know that as there is a Mother Earth, there is a Father Heaven. Many people in the spiritual practice always want to raise themselves to a higher level to be filled with spiritual energy. If you want to go higher, you must take care that the foundation, the rooting, is good. This connection of heaven and earth is most important in the Tao practice. In the higher practice, the ground energy from Mother Earth is equally important to the spiritual energy from Father Heaven.

To assist you at this point with an overall view of the Embracing the Tree posture, see Figure 3–10(a) through (g).

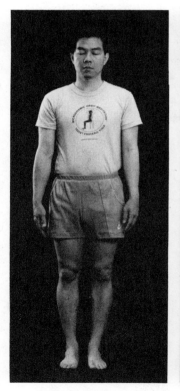 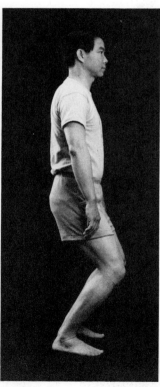 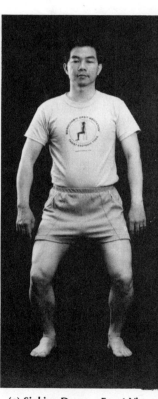

(a) Beginning Posture   (b) Sinking Down—Side View   (c) Sinking Down—Front View

FIGURE 3–10

Embracing the Tree Posture

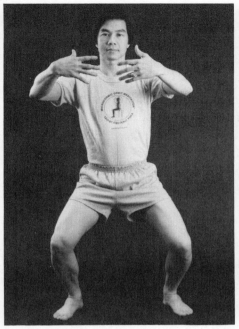

(d) Full Embracing the Tree Posture—Front View

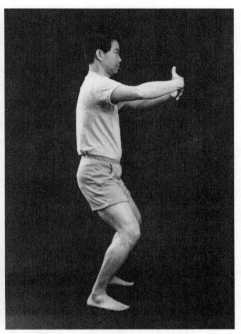

(e) Full Embracing the Tree Posture—Side View

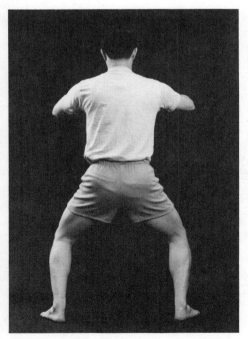

(f) Full Embracing the Tree Posture—Back View

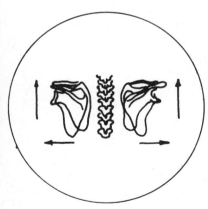

(g) Rounding of the Scapulae

3. Elongation of the Spine (Figure 3–11(a), (b) and (c))

When you feel the CHI and fullness down below the navel, slowly sink down into the knees and feel the sacrum pulling the spine down and the head stretching upward as if pulled by a string. Keep the spine erect. Feel the spine suspended upward and the sacrum downward in order to help elongate the spine and keep the discs released. Gradually you will become taller. This elongation gives more room for expansion of the nervous system and for spinal fluid and CHI to travel freely. Look straight ahead, and step to the side with the left foot to the standard position.

Feel the head stretch up as if pulled by a string

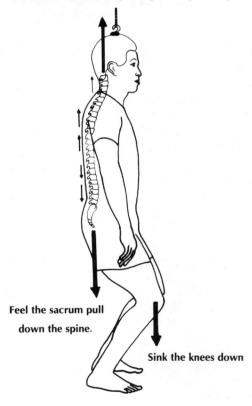

Feel the sacrum pull down the spine.

Sink the knees down

FIGURE 3-11

(a) Elongation of the Spine

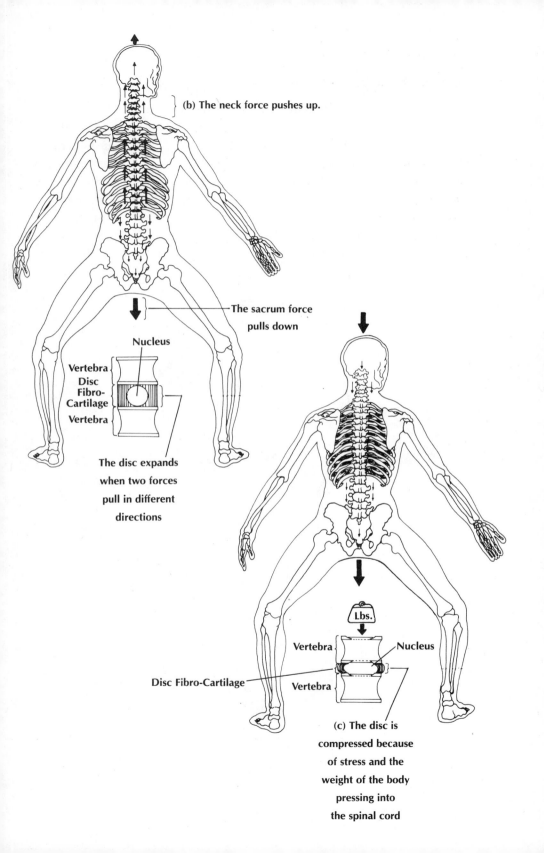

(b) The neck force pushes up.

The sacrum force pulls down

Nucleus

Vertebra
Disc
Fibro-
Cartilage
Vertebra

The disc expands
when two forces
pull in different
directions

Lbs.

Vertebra — Nucleus

Disc Fibro-Cartilage

Vertebra

(c) The disc is
compressed because
of stress and the
weight of the body
pressing into
the spinal cord

4. Three CHI Circles

a. Connect the arm with the scapula—the First Circle (Figure 3–12)

Raise your arms in a circle as if holding a large ball or a tree lightly between the hands and chest. This forms the first circle. Your fingers should be gently separated by holding the fingertips of each hand one to two inches apart from each other. The neck (C–7) is the main juncture where energy and the powerful tendons of the body meet. Gradually you will feel the CHI spread from the C–7 to the outside of the arm, to the middle finger, to the palm and feel the CHI jump from the right middle finger to the left middle finger, and from the right thumb to the left thumb.

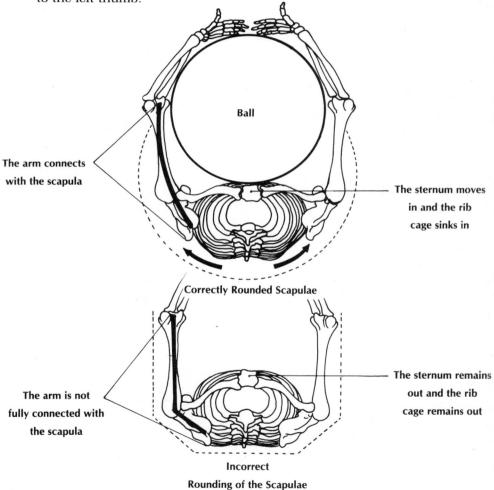

FIGURE 3-12

The First Circle: Connect the arms with the scapulae

Elbows sink down, turning inward, and should feel as if they are maintaining their position by resisting the downward pull. Imagine that someone is pushing you on the outside of your elbows and you, in turn, are pushing outward to maintain the position. Feel the spiral in your forearm as if it were a screw turning clockwise. This will connect the wrist, elbow and arm together. Relax the shoulders. Drop the neck muscles down. The trapezius muscles, connecting the back of the neck with the back of the shoulders, have to be relaxed so that the connection can be transformed down. (Figure 3–13) Bring your concentration down the spine, pressing down on your skeletal structure to the sacrum, to the knees, and finally down to the feet and the

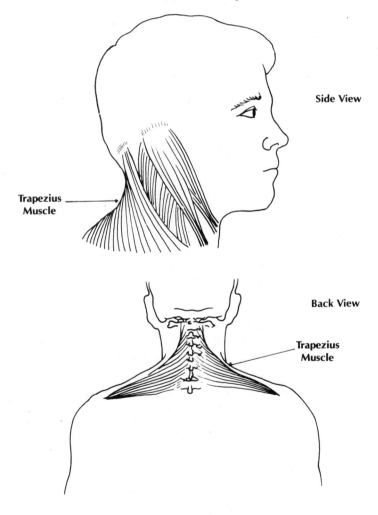

Side View

**Trapezius
Muscle**

Back View

**Trapezius
Muscle**

FIGURE 3-13

Trapezius Muscle

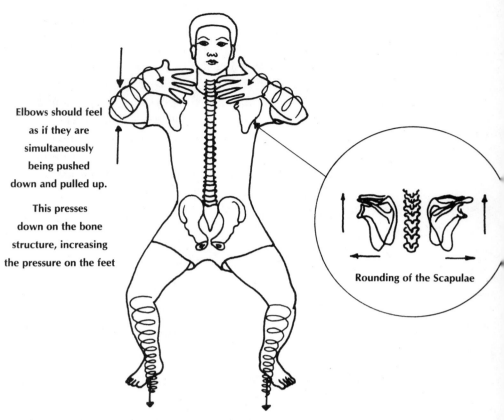

Elbows should feel as if they are simultaneously being pushed down and pulled up.

This presses down on the bone structure, increasing the pressure on the feet

Rounding of the Scapulae

Feet press down through pressure on the bone structure.

FIGURE 3-14

Press down on the bone structure

earth. You are pressing down on the skeletal structure for the body's support, rather than the muscles. The pressure gradually travels down the spine to the sacrum and hips, tightening the legs and feet. Eventually you will feel your bone structure connected down to the ground, rooted as if you had grown into the ground and were all one piece with the earth. (Figure 3-14)

Stand erect, feet close together, and feel the weight distributed evenly on the feet. Relax the neck, the shoulders and the chest. Gradually bring your attention to the navel and send the CHI energy to the navel until you feel a warm fullness there.

b. Connect the scapulae with the spine—the Second Circle

(Figure 3–15(a), (b) and (c))

Thumbs point up so that the energy will flow between the two thumbs and the energy will connect with the big toes; thus, the two muscle-tendon meridians join together, and the front structure of bones, tendons, fasciae and muscles tighten the structure together as one. (Figure 3–15(a))

Attach the hands and fingers to the scapulae, or shoulder blades,

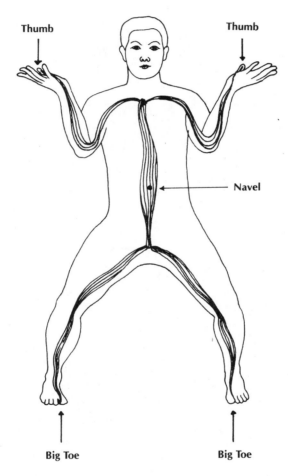

(a) Feel the thumbs' lines and big toes' lines connect. Their union will help join the front body structure

FIGURE 3-15

The Second Circle: Connect the scapulae with the spine   99

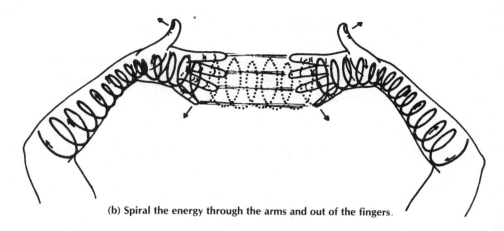

(b) Spiral the energy through the arms and out of the fingers.

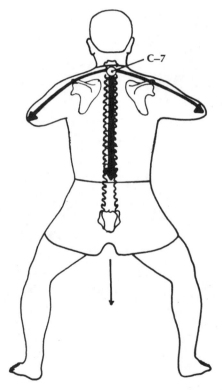

C–7

(c) Stretch like a bow from C–7 to the thumbs, thereby connecting the hands,
C-7, scapulae and spine

FIGURE 3-15

and cranial bone by pulling the thumb tendons away from the body and the pinky fingers' tendons towards you. Feel a spiraling action turning in a clockwise circle as you pull the scapulae to the side. (Figure 3–15(b)) As in using the wall, feel as though the inner edges of the shoulder blades remain on the wall with the shoulder blades sticking to the back of the rib cage. This will allow the transference of force from the shoulder blades to the rib cage, which in turn will transfer to the C–7, or energy junction point, to the spine, the sacrum, the knees and down to the feet. In this way the force can also be transferred from the earth to the feet, to the knees, to the hips, to the sacrum, to the spine, to the shoulder blades and, finally, to the hands. Since the shoulder blades, while near the spine, are not connected to it, there can be no force transferred from one to the other unless you practice the proper stretching.

In practicing this posture, you will feel a stretch of force form like a bow from C–7 to the thumb. When your elbows sink and press inward, you will feel more of the stretching of the bow. By stretching the scapulae and spine tendons and connecting them together (Figure 3–15(c)), the back becomes rounded and the chest sinks. Feel the hollowness of the chest. The sternum then sinks down to press the thymus gland, the major gland of rejuvenation and the immune system. (Figure 3–16) Keeping this gland active will increase CHI flow.

These events will help to activate the cranial pump. (Figure 3–17) Rest and feel the head start to pulsate. Joining the powerful muscle-tendon meridian down to the navel will connect the CHI energy in the front line and join the bone structure of the rib cage together. (Figure 3–15(a)) In doing so you are helping to sink the energy down. This forms the Second Circle.

Embracing the Tree will strengthen the thumb and toe muscles and tendons along this meridian. The thumb and toes have the principal rooting power.

By strengthening these muscles tendon meridians which join at the navel, all the muscles, tendons, bones and fasciae (connective tissues) will become tied together, greatly improving the bone structure and holding a good posture.

Bad posture is caused by weak tendons, muscles and fasciae, which cause bones to fall easily out of alignment.

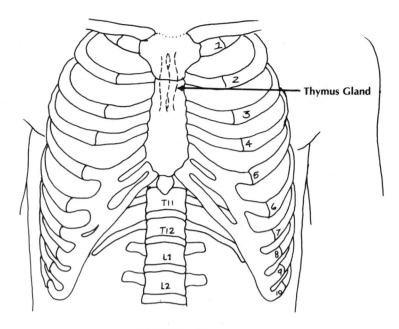

FIGURE 3-16

The Thymus Gland is the major gland of rejuvenation and the immune system

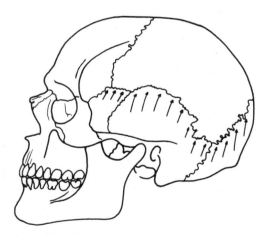

The Cranial Pump becomes activated during the Second Circle when, upon deep inhalation, there is a micromovement of the Cranial Bones

FIGURE 3-17

The Cranial Pump

c. Connect the hand, scapulae and spine to the sacrum—the Third Circle (Figure 3–18)

This connection is made by pushing out the curve of the C–7 from the sternum, the natural curve of the spine, and locking the hips. This will stretch the spine like a flexed bow that will link the spine, C–7, scapulae, shoulders, arms, elbows, and hands together. Push the sacrum out as if you were pushing against the wall; the hips remain the same. The hip bones and sacrum can be separated individually. Once you can separate out and move the sacrum straight, you can activitate the sacral pump which is very important to help circulate the CHI.

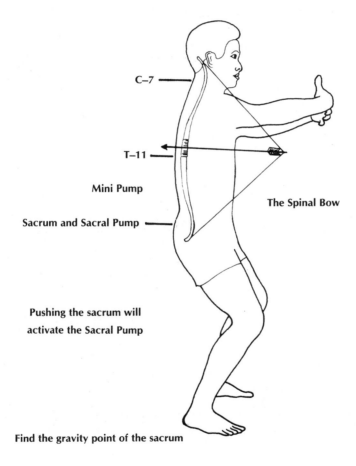

FIGURE 3-18

The Third Circle: Connect the hands, scapulae and spine to the sacrum

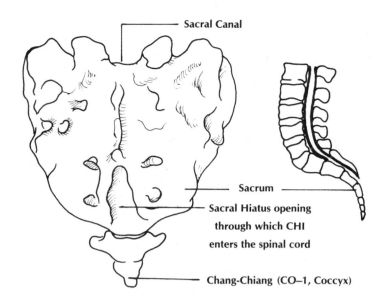

Sacral Canal

Sacrum

Sacral Hiatus opening
through which CHI
enters the spinal cord

Chang-Chiang (CO–1, Coccyx)

FIGURE 3-19

The Sacral Pump

(Figure 3–19) You will feel the connection of the spine, the scapulae and the sacrum. Find and adjust the gravity point of the sacrum in between the feet.

The greatest kinetic energy and power in the human body is generated through the hip joints, around which are attached the largest muscles (the psoas muscles). (Figure 3–20) However, if you cannot open the pelvis and differentiate both sides (pelvic differentiation), the power of the hip joints is limited to only two directions. The simple fact of standing on one leg without leaning to one side would require an internal sense of the angle of the pelvis, and the arrangement of the spine. To feel "empty" on one side can only happen when you feel grounded, supported and aligned on the other (emptiness and fullness: Yin-Yang).

Round the pelvic area like an arched bow. By turning the big toes in slightly, the second toes point straight ahead so that your feet are positioned as though standing on the circumference of a circle, making yet another circle. This will gradually open the groin area and allow the CHI pressure to fill the area as if a ball were in this area.

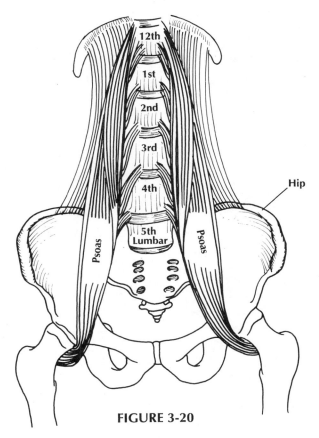

FIGURE 3-20

Opening the Pelvic Area

The hip joints are synergistically dependent upon two further joint alignments: the knees and ankles.

The knees, ankles and feet are the next connection to the earth. Embracing the Tree requires a precise alignment of the knee and ankle joints. The critical joint alignment is in the "saddle" of the tibia (shin bone) over the talus (ankle bone), which stabilizes everything above. Sink down and open the knees a little bit, turning the knees outward slightly as if you were in a saddle. Feel a spiraling downward movement as if your legs were screws, screwing down into the ground, created by pressing firmly on the feet, and then feel the whole

105

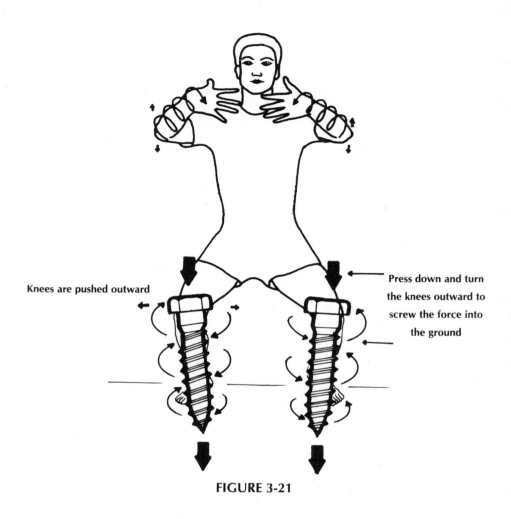

Knees are pushed outward

Press down and turn the knees outward to screw the force into the ground

FIGURE 3-21

Screw the force into the ground

body force transfer to the ankles, the feet, and to the ground. (Figure 3–21) Feel your bone structure. The knees should feel as if they are simultaneously being pushed in and out. Lock the knee caps.

If the alignment is oblique, forces through the feet are not spread evenly.

The knee joints should not be positioned over the big toes as this may cause some to experience knee pain, making them unable to continue. If you have trouble with your knees while in the Horse Stance, you must judge just how much you can do. In your own best interest,

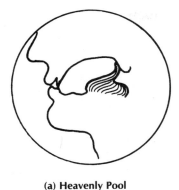 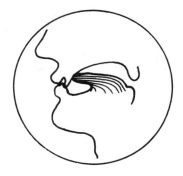

(a) Heavenly Pool　　　　　　　　(b) The tongue touches behind the teeth

FIGURE 3-22

Tongue Positions

you may have to forego some of the positions. Note, however, that the cause of pain is not necessarily found in the physical location in which the pain is felt.

Fold the tongue back to the soft palate in the area of the Heavenly Pool. (Figure 3–22(a)) If this is difficult, simply touch the tip of the tongue to the gum line behind the front upper teeth. (Figure 3–22(b)) Now you should feel the whole body structure connect into one piece from the feet, ankles, knees, hips, sacrum, spinal cord, scapulae, arms, elbows and hands.

5. The Eyes Can Help to Direct CHI

The Taoists regard the eyes as the windows of the soul and a most powerful tool in directing and absorbing CHI into the body.

Direct the eyes to look at the fingertips of both hands. Hold the eyes steady to direct the CHI flow. Keep them wide open while looking at the fingertips to help connect the CHI between the fingers while seeing the tip of your nose with some part of your vision. Allow the ears to listen inside the body to the navel. (Figure 3–23) This will make you feel very centered, peaceful and calm.

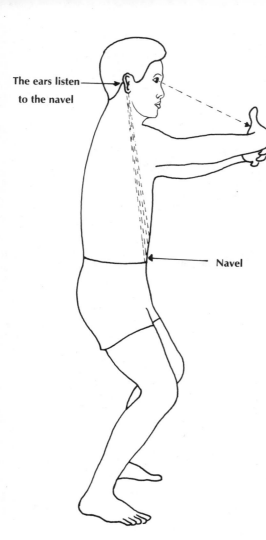

The ears listen to the navel

Navel

FIGURE 3-23

During inhalation, create a ball by expanding the abdomen on all sides
Exhale and feel the ball roll up your chest

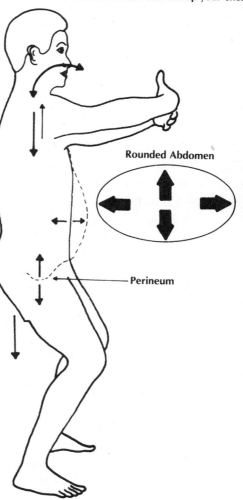

Rounded Abdomen

Perineum

FIGURE 3-24

Energizer Breathing

6. Begin with Energizer Breathing (Abdominal and Reverse Breathing)

Concentrate on the area just one and one-half inches inside and below the navel until you feel some CHI activity there. At that point, begin breathing, preferably the Energizer Breathing. As described in Chapter 2, this is accomplished by first inhaling into the lower abdomen (the region below the navel). Feel the abdominal wall pull the lower lobes of the lungs down and the air move in. Feel the lower abdomen and perineum bulge on all sides like a ball, then forcibly expel the air through your nostrils. With this expulsion of air, feel as if a ball were rolling up your chest. (Figure 3–24) Sink the sternum and press into the thymus gland. At the same time, pull up the sex organs and the anus. When exhaling, the abdomen is flat to the spine. Release. One such inhalation and exhalation constitutes a round.

7. First Stage

a. Do nine to eighteen rounds of Energizer Breathing. Remember, the breath should be generated from the lower abdomen, one and one-half inches below the navel. You can put your hand at the lower abdominal area to make sure the breathing is generating from there.

b. Exhale your last inhalation and be aware of how you flatten the abdomen, pulling in and up behind the front lower ribs to do this. This will increase and strengthen the psoas muscle. Exhale once more and relax the diaphragm downwards. Gradually you will feel the diaphragm press against the adrenal gland. (Figure 3–25) Do not tighten the abdomen. Contract the perineum and start to do the Iron Shirt Packing Process.

c. Perineum power: Inhale ten percent of your capacity with short, quick breaths generating from the navel by using the navel to pull the air in and pull up the sexual organs. (Men pull up the testicles and the penis; women pull up the uterus and squeeze the vagina tight.) Keep the abdominals in the position they assumed when you exhaled and feel pressure build in the upper abdomen. (Figure 3–26)

d. Inhale another ten percent and pull up the left side of the anus. Bring the CHI to the left kidney and wrap and pack the kidney and adrenal glands with CHI. (Figure 3–27) In the beginning you might not feel it, but when you practice for a while, you will feel something

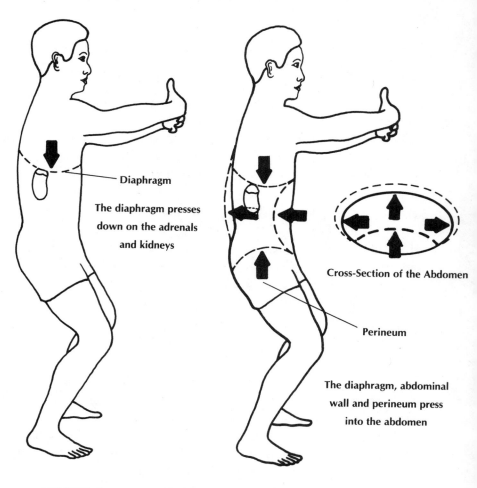

FIGURE 3-25

Relax the diaphragm downwards

Diaphragm

The diaphragm presses
down on the adrenals
and kidneys

Cross-Section of the Abdomen

Perineum

The diaphragm, abdominal
wall and perineum press
into the abdomen

FIGURE 3-26

Perineum Power

under the back rib cage bulge out. The sensation is very unusual. Inhale again to the right side of the anus and pull the CHI to wrap
around the right kidney. The kidneys are the first organs to be exercised. Remember, the first point of each kidney, K–1, is on the sole of
each foot; these points are the major points of rooting. When the kidneys are strong, the bones will be strong because the kidneys control
the bones and the CHI in the bones. When you can master the kidneys' Packing Process, that is, wrapping and packing the CHI around
the kidneys, you can easily move to wrapping and packing the ovaries,

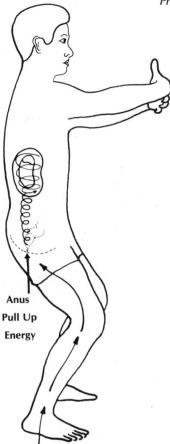

FIGURE 3-27

Wrap the energy around the kidneys

prostate gland, adrenal glands, liver, spleen, lungs, heart, and thymus gland. (Figure 3–28)

e. Concentrate on the navel and circle the CHI in that area nine times in a clockwise direction in an area three inches in diameter, and nine times in a counterclockwise direction, thereby condensing the CHI into a ball. (Figure 3–29) Use your mind and eye movements to help create the circular direction by moving the eyes in a round circle. (Figure 3–30) First move the eyes clockwise beginning with the eyes looking downward, moving up to the right corner, to the top, to

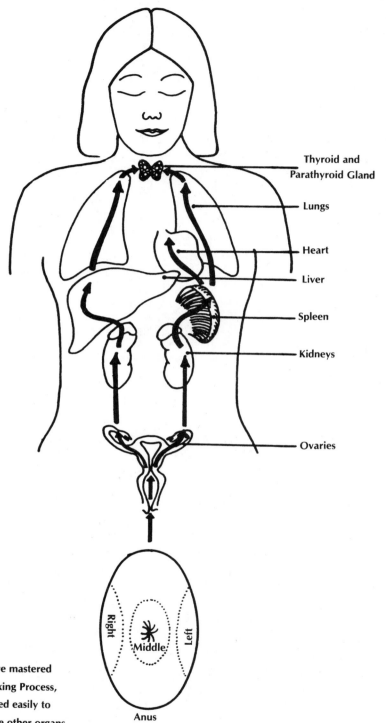

Thyroid and
Parathyroid Gland

Lungs

Heart

Liver

Spleen

Kidneys

Ovaries

Once you have mastered
the kidney Packing Process,
you can proceed easily to
wrap and pack the other organs

Right

Middle

Left

Anus

FIGURE 3-28

The Kidney Packing Process

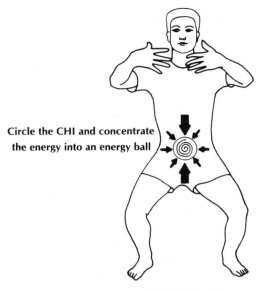

Circle the CHI and concentrate the energy into an energy ball

FIGURE 3-29

Creating an Energy Ball

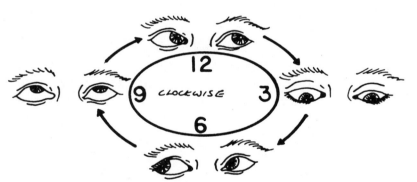

Use the mind and eyes to help circle the CHI energy ball nine times
clockwise . . . and nine times counterclockwise

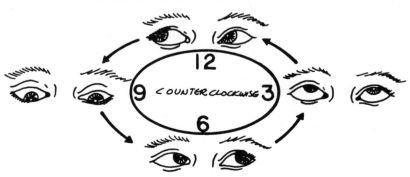

FIGURE 3-30

Circulate the energy ball

the left corner and down again **nine** times; then, circulate the CHI counterclockwise by moving the eyes from the bottom to the left, to the top, down to the right, and to the bottom nine times.

You should begin at your navel and circle inwards using a three inch diameter, while thinking that the CHI in the body is being drawn to that place by that activity and that it is being packed into the smaller and smaller area of an energy ball, to be finally contained in the navel. Slowly do nine rounds. Concentrate and collect your energy when you feel CHI has been generated. The CHI will condense into a small, dense unit.

There are nine points in which the CHI is to be circulated and condensed. (Figure 3–64) In later practice, you will condense, store and bring up the CHI from these power stations. These CHI power stations are tremendously useful in the Kung Fu energy and spiritual practice.

It is most important to keep the diaphram down. Remember to check it by touching the sternum and the stomach. You can feel the diaphram coming down when it is distinguishable from the stomach.

f. Inhale another ten percent. If you feel that you cannot inhale more, you can exhale very little and inhale again. Make the abdomen flatter and draw CHI into the lower abdominal area. The area below the navel seems to be filled, but keep the upper abdomen flat in order to minimize the space so that the CHI pressure can be increased. As mentioned previously, this sensation is caused by the action of the diaphragm pressing down against the organs contained in the abdomen. The pressure between the outer wall of muscle of the abdomen, which is kept flat, and that of the diaphragm pushing down from above serves to compress the abdominal organs. When you pull up the pelvic and urogenital diaphram and pull up the sex organs and anus, more energy will pack in the lower abdominal area. There is where the CHI is condensed into an energy ball. This energy ball will expel wastes and rinse out the toxins from the system, aiding in the circulation of blood and lymph through the area and driving excess CHI into storage between the fascial layers. (Figure 3–31) Remember, the CHI will occupy this space, prohibiting fat from being stored there.

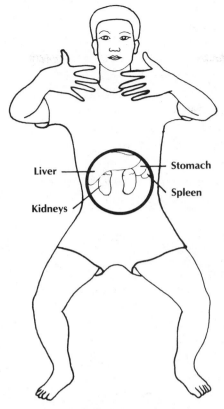

Liver — Stomach

Spleen

Kidneys

Packing and condensing the organs will help to expel
toxins and wastes from the body

FIGURE 3-31

Pack and condense the organs

g. Inhaling ten percent more of your total capacity presses the diaphragm even lower, so that now you become more aware of the contents of the lower abdominal area. (Figure 3–32(a)) Women should be aware of the area in which the ovaries rest. Hold your breath until the need arises to inhale.

It is at this point that you can work on your feet and coccyx, which are most important as energy sources. Those who have already completed the Microcosmic Orbit should make rapid progress here.

h. Inhale ten percent more of your capacity. Concentration should now be on the sexual organs.

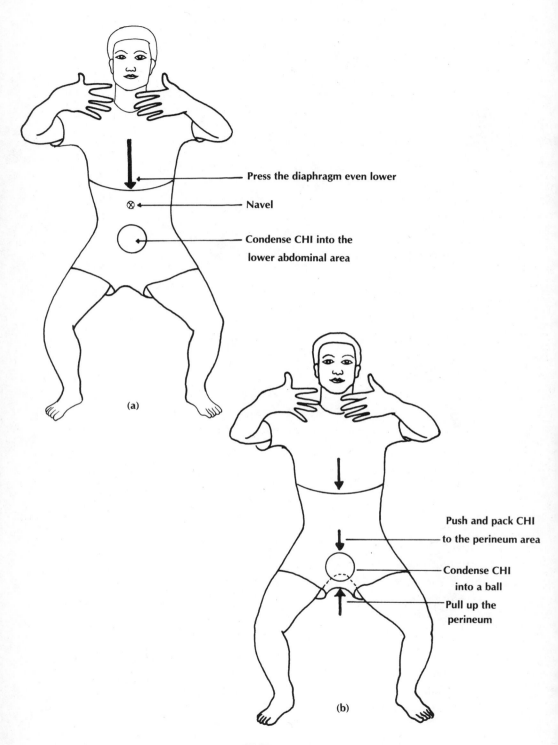

Press the diaphragm even lower

Navel

Condense CHI into the
lower abdominal area

(a)

Push and pack CHI
to the perineum area

Condense CHI
into a ball

Pull up the
perineum

(b)

FIGURE 3–32

Condensing CHI

With more practice your mind can direct the CHI more easily, giving you greater control over the CHI energy. Condense the CHI into a compact ball. Hold this energy in the lower abdominal area where you can increase it by using your mind and the Packing Process.

i. Inhale ten percent more of your capacity to the Hui Yin (perineum) to activate Perineum Power. Pull up the perineum, push and pack the CHI down to the perineum area and condense it into a ball. (Figure 3–32(b)) Concentrate on the perineum again. With more practice you will gradually feel the perineum bulge downward. You should be able to feel a big channel running from the navel to the abdomen to the perineum connecting with CHI. Hold the breath as long as you feel comfortable.

j. Now, exhale and relax the whole body, sending energy down the back of the legs into the ground. (Figure 3–33) Regulate your breathing

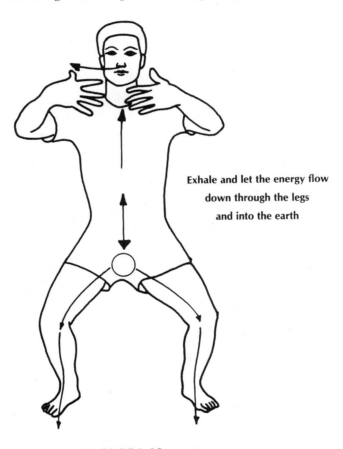

Exhale and let the energy flow
down through the legs
and into the earth

FIGURE 3-33

Send the energy into the earth

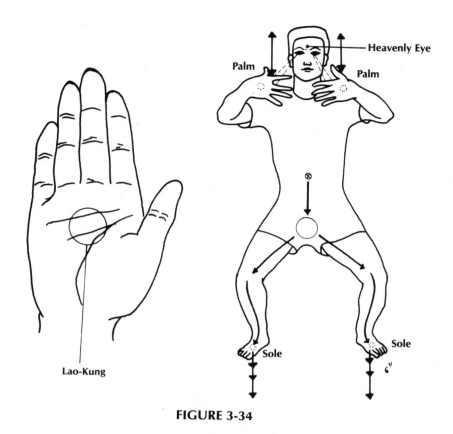

FIGURE 3-34

Feel the palms and soles breathing

with energizer breathing. Inhale more; exhale less. When you exhale, pull up the perineum (include the sex organs and anus). Be aware of the middle of the palms of the hands and the middle of the soles of the feet. Use the mind to feel the palms and soles "breathing". Coordinate your breath with the palms and soles, breathing simultaneously. With the Packing Process Breathing, the palms and soles will open easily. Gradually, you will feel as though the soles and palms seem to breathe. (Figure 3–34) The left eye looks at the left palm, the right eye looks at the right palm. In the forehead, above and between the eyebrows, resides what the Taoists regard as another eye called the "Heavenly Eye". Feel the CHI from the palms flow to the forehead while the "Heavenly Eye" sends CHI to the palms.

Now, exhale and relax the whole body, bringing the CHI down the backs of the legs to the soles of the feet and hold your attention there.

Concentrate on the soles until you feel the energy going down into the ground. Gradually, increase the energy down to the ground and feel as though you are growing roots like the roots of a tree inch-by-inch downward, at first six inches, then one foot, and so on. Feel the flow of CHI from the navel to the perineum, to the backs of the knees, to the soles of the feet and down into the ground. Become one line of energy flow.

k. When you can feel that you are rooting into the earth, you are hooking up to Mother Earth's inexhaustible sources of energy. (Figure 3–35) Become aware of the "loving, healing energy" emanating from

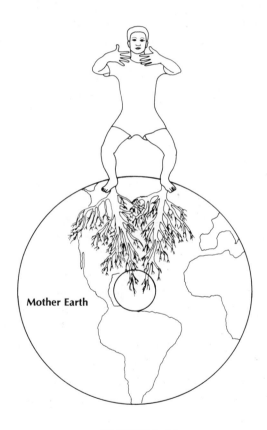

FIGURE 3-35

Hooking up to Mother Earth's inexhaustible sources of energy

Mother Earth, which enters through the soles and rises up the front of the legs six inches at first, then two feet, then three feet or more. Continue in this way until your whole body is full of this "loving, healing energy". Hold and pack the CHI in the perineum until you feel the urge to breathe. Exhale and do the Energizing Breathing to regulate your breath.

At the end of each stage, once you have finished packing the CHI, standing or holding yourself still and relaxing the muscles of the whole body are very important. You should hold this position for as long as you can or have time to hold it, gradually increasing the time, if possible. Using the Iron Shirt Chi Kung Packing Breathing has created a tremendous CHI pressure and you can now use your mind to condense and direct the flow. (Figure 3–36) At this point, you will fully

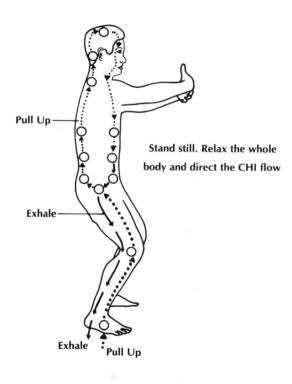

Pull Up

Stand still. Relax the whole body and direct the CHI flow

Exhale

Exhale   Pull Up

FIGURE 3-36

Direct the CHI flow

feel the energy flow in the Microcosmic Orbit. Use your mind to direct the energy up and down, flowing from finger to finger, down the legs and back up.

In the beginning it seems that you are very tense and nervous when you practice Iron Shirt, the way you felt when first learning to ride a bicycle. However, once you are trained and know how to move and pack the energy, you use more structure and mind control with confidence and less muscle.

Each time you finish a stage and are not proceeding to the next stage, you must collect the CHI in the navel. Stand up straight, touch the tongue to the palate, and put the palms over the navel. Men put the right palm over the navel, covering it with the left palm. Women put the left palm over the navel, covering it with the right palm.

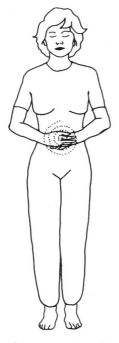
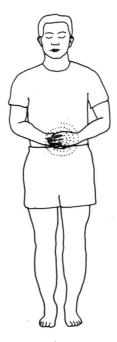

The woman places the
right palm over the left

The man places the
left palm over the right

FIGURE 3-37

Place the palm over the navel and collect the CHI

121

(Figure 3–37) Concentrate on the navel for a while, feeling the energy that is generated by the Chi Kung. As you are standing, practice the Bone Breathing Process described below.

Practice the first stage for a week or two, until you can master moving the CHI from the navel to K–1 at the soles of the feet and master palm and sole breathing, and then proceed on.

8. Second Stage

Begin with the First Stage and continue as follows:

a. Press the soles of the feet to the floor so that they seem to adhere to it by suction. The toes are part of a tendon line and, as such, are part of an energy flow line. To take advantage of this fact, press and clamp all of the toes firmly to the floor, but do not allow them to bulge up. When concentrating on the soles, you may find that they grow warm or feel cool. Inhale ten percent and coordinate with the breath, sucking the earth energy into your soles. Inhale ten percent using the Packing Process Breathing technique described in the First Stage. (Figure 3–38) Pull the energy up to the sexual organs and the urogenital

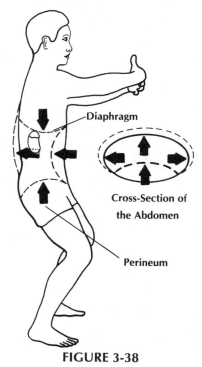

Diaphragm

Cross-Section of
the Abdomen

Perineum

FIGURE 3-38

Pull and lower the entire diaphragm

diaphragm, the pelvic diaphragm, the left and right anus, the kidneys (Figure 3–39) and the lower diaphragm. Feel as though you are sucking the earth. Feel the earth energy begin to enter the soles and move up the leg bones to the knees. The earth energy can feel cool or sometimes tingling. Some people feel warm.

b. Using your K–1 center in the soles of the feet as a hub, circle nine times clockwise out from the middle to a distance of three inches, and then nine times counterclockwise back to K–1. (Figure 3–40) Again, use the mind, coordinating with eye movements, to help circulate the energy.

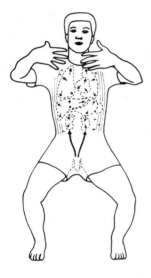

FIGURE 3-39

Pull the energy up from the anus to the kidneys

Inhale ten percent and press the soles of the feet firmly into the earth Claw the toes and circulate the energy nine times

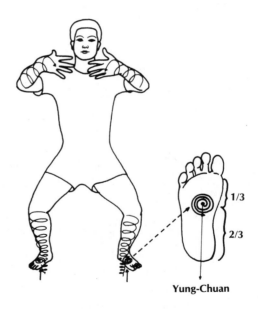

1/3

2/3

Yung-Chuan

FIGURE 3-40

Use the K–1 center in the soles of the feet as a hub

123

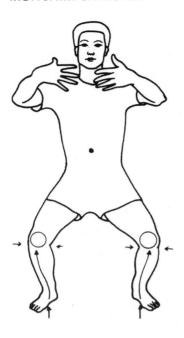
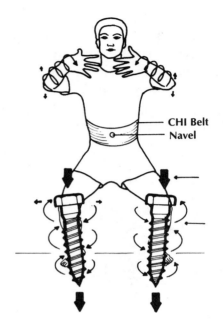

CHI Belt
Navel

(a) Inhale twenty percent
and bring the energy up to the
knees. Lock the knees

(b) Press down and turn
the knees outward to
screw the force into
the ground

FIGURE 3-41

Screw the force into the ground

c. Inhale and bring the energy up out of the big toes to the knees. Lock the knee cap and tighten the legs by turning the knees outward with the feet firm. (Figure 3–41(a)) Feel the legs like screws being screwed into the ground. (Figure 3–41(b)) Imagine someone pushing the knees in while you try to push outward. Slightly pull the knees outward and feel the outside force push in. This action will join the sacrum with the knees, and the knees with the ankles and the feet. This also activates and aligns all the lower part tendons together. Remember that the feet point in, and the knees push slightly outward.

Concentrate on them until you feel energy collect there. Do not circulate the energy at this point.

When you feel the urge to breathe, you can exhale a little bit. Exhaling and inhaling are very personalized; therefore, each person must adjust to his or her own needs.

d. (1) Inhale ten percent, coordinating the breath with pulling in the sexual organs and anus, thereby bringing the energy up your knees to the buttocks and then to the perineum (Hui Yin). At the same time, feel the energy as it is drawn from the earth enter the soles of the feet and rise to the knees and perineum. Inhale and pack more in the perineum. Use your eyes to help circulate the CHI energy nine times clockwise and nine times counterclockwise in a three inch diameter at the perineum. (Figure 3–42)

Increasingly send energy down to the Hui Yin from the navel, and

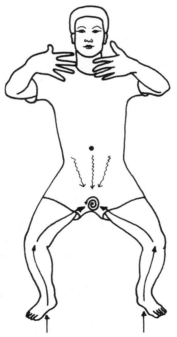

Pull the sexual organs and anus in. Inhale ten percent up to the perineum

Circulate the energy nine times clockwise and nine times counterclockwise

FIGURE 3-42

Draw the energy from the earth
and pack and circulate it in the perineum

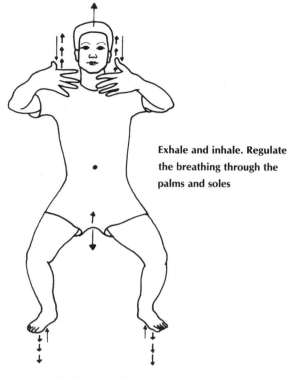

Exhale and inhale. Regulate the breathing through the palms and soles

FIGURE 3-43

Energizer Breathing

continue to feel it come up out of the legs. In time, it may seem as though there is a flow, as of water, entering the Hui Yin from above and from below, moving up and down as though through a pipe. It might also become evident why the K–1 points in the soles of the feet are referred to as the "Bubbling Springs".

(2) Exhale and normalize the breath by Energizing Breathing. (Figure 3–43) Relax and collect "loving energy" from all of the organs. To create the loving energy, you can start your smile in the eyes. Bring that smile down the face, slightly lifting the corner of the mouth, and keep on smiling inwardly to the organs: the heart, lungs, liver, pancreas, spleen, kidneys and sexual organs. (Figure 3–44)

Remember, standing or holding yourself still at this point and re-

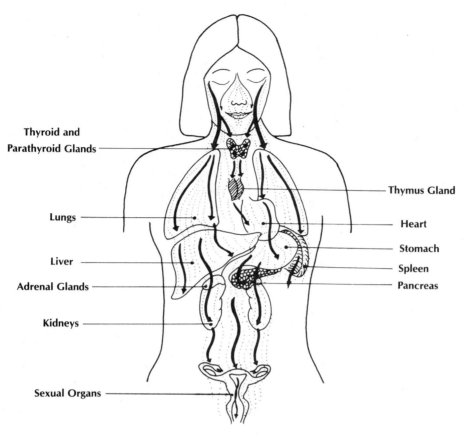

FIGURE 3-44

Smile down to the organs

laxing the muscles of the whole body are very important. Feel the energy flow in the Microcosmic Orbit. (Figure 3–45) Remember also that after each stage, if you are not proceeding to the next stage, you must collect the CHI in the navel. Stand up straight, touch the tongue to the palate, and put the palms over the navel. Men put the right palm over the navel, covering it with the left palm. Women put the left palm over the navel, covering it with the right palm. (Figure 3–46) Concentrate on the navel for a while, feeling the energy that is generated by the Chi Kung. As you are standing, practice the Bone Breathing Process described below.

which has just been described above as the First and Second Stages. Proceed to the next stage.

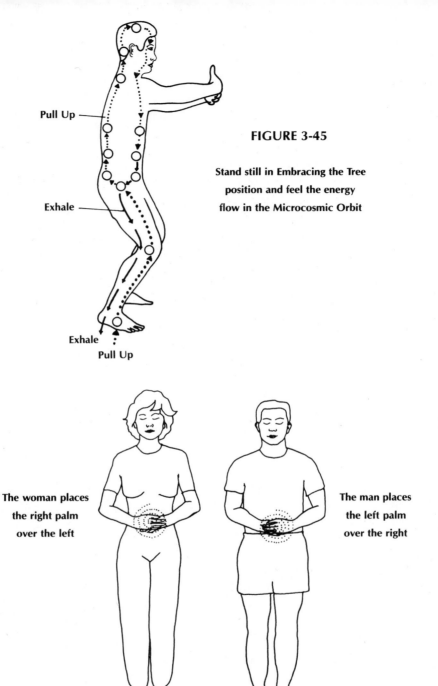

FIGURE 3-45

Stand still in Embracing the Tree
position and feel the energy
flow in the Microcosmic Orbit

Pull Up

Exhale

Exhale

Pull Up

The woman places
the right palm
over the left

The man places
the left palm
over the right

FIGURE 3-46

Place the palms over the navel to collect the energy

9. Third Stage

Begin by repeating the First and Second Stages, then proceed as follows:

a. After you have normalized the breath, exhale and flatten the stomach. Inhale ten percent using the Packing Process Breathing as described in the First Stage. Inhale up the front and middle of the anus, and at the same time, pull up the back part of the anus so that you can direct the CHI into the sacrum. (Figure 3–47(a) and (b)) Put

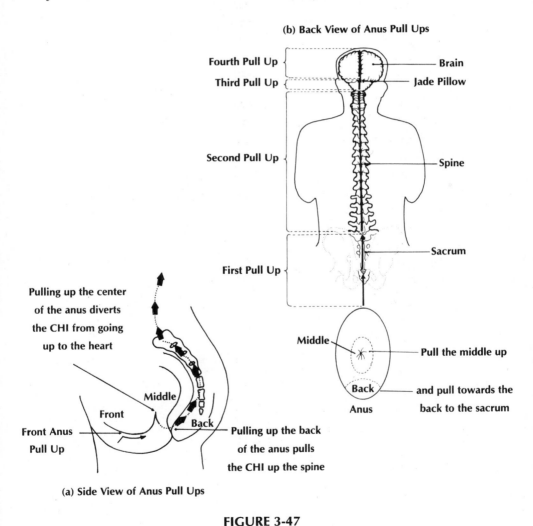

(b) Back View of Anus Pull Ups

Fourth Pull Up — Brain
Third Pull Up — Jade Pillow
Second Pull Up — Spine
— Sacrum
First Pull Up

Pulling up the center of the anus diverts the CHI from going up to the heart

Middle — Pull the middle up
Back — and pull towards the
Anus — back to the sacrum

Middle
Front
Back
Front Anus Pull Up — Pulling up the back of the anus pulls the CHI up the spine

(a) Side View of Anus Pull Ups

FIGURE 3-47

Direct the CHI into the sacrum

pressure on the sacrum by pressing tightly to the ground and tilting the sacrum back without moving the hips. This will activate the sacral pump. (Figure 3–48) You can practice this by putting your back to the wall and pressing the sacrum to touch the wall, as described in Section I of this Chapter. Do this gradually and do not force it. In gradually developing the psoas muscle, as well as the hip and sacrum tendons and muscles, you will be able to move the sacrum separately. (Figure 3–49) By this movement, you are activating the sacral pump to help increase the spinal fluid and to open the sacrum for the CHI to enter. This will greatly increase the circulation of spinal fluid. When you can master this, you will no longer need the wall. Use wall alignment in practicing Embracing the Tree.

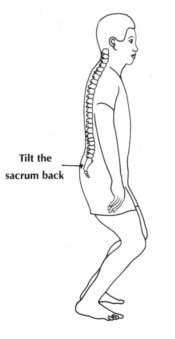

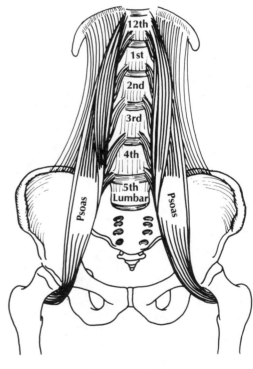

FIGURE 3-48

Activate the
sacral pump

FIGURE 3-49

The sacral tilt will help
develop the psoas muscle

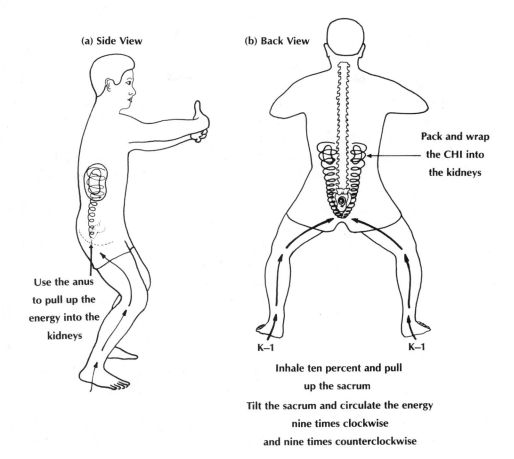

(a) Side View

(b) Back View

Pack and wrap
the CHI into
the kidneys

Use the anus
to pull up the
energy into the
kidneys

K–1   K–1

Inhale ten percent and pull
up the sacrum

Tilt the sacrum and circulate the energy
nine times clockwise
and nine times counterclockwise

FIGURE 3-50

Pack and wrap the CHI into the kidneys.

b. (1) Bring more energy (kidneys' energy) up from K–1 on the soles of the feet to the coccyx and to the sacrum. Inhale, pulling up the left and right anus and the back part of the anus. Pull up toward the coccyx and up to the sacrum, packing CHI to the kidneys. (Figure 3–50(a)) Feel the back area surrounding the kidneys bulge out. Concentrating here, tilt the sacrum and circle the energy out at the sacrum from that point first nine times clockwise to a distance of three inches, and then nine times counterclockwise back to the sacrum, using the eyes to help direct the circulation. (Figure 3–50(b)) Feel the collection of the CHI there.

The CHI feeling is reported differently, even by the same practitioner at different times. There can be a range of feelings such as hot or cold, or pricklings, vibrations, numbness or a combination of all of these and other sensations. The effect is identifiable as something which is not ordinarily experienced. There might be pain or extremes of sensation. This part of the practice should take one or two weeks.

I feel that it is necessary to stress that in this system you must realize that what you experience is very real. There are no visualizations or acts of the imagination here. You actually feel energy accumulate and then go from place to place because it really does. In some people it takes off on its own and goes through the very same routes and stopping off places that would have later been prescribed. If this happens to you, it is extremely convincing and is thereafter self-evident that there really is CHI and that all one needs to do is follow.

(2) When you feel CHI in the sacrum, inhale ten percent and pull the CHI up to T–11, tilting the T–11 (the adrenal glands, CHI-Chung, CO–6) back. (Figure 3-51(a)) This will push the lower back and straighten the curve. Again, use the wall as a guide. Do not force your spine, but gently ease it until you feel the spine becoming straight. This will open the Door of Life Center (Lumbar 2 and Lumbar 3) opposite the navel. The pumping action will increase as the spine straightens, pulling like a pipe or bow, and the CHI will flow easily as if through a straight pipe. With the lower back pushed and the curve straightened, you will be stretching the psoas muscle very strongly. This will help to strengthen the lower back tremendously. Connect the sacrum and the C–7 into one pipe or a bow. Bring the CHI to T–11, concentrating at this center, and circle the CHI outward clockwise to a distance of three inches. Do this nine times and then circle back nine times down to that center in a counterclockwise direction, finally concentrating it there. (Figure 3–51(b)) It can take you from less than a week to more than three weeks to develop to the point where the sacrum and the T–11 fuse into one channel.

It is important to remember that each time you start to inhale and pack, you must start at the navel, gather the CHI, and bring the energy gathered there to the Hui Yin. Then, push the energy to the ground. Bring it up from the soles to the Hui Yin, and mix it with the energy already brought down from the navel before going on to the coccyx,

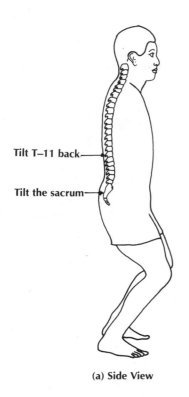

Tilt T–11 back

Tilt the sacrum

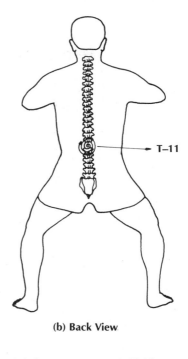

T–11

(b) Back View

(a) Side View

Inhale ten percent up to T–11.

Tilt T–11 back and circulate the energy nine times clockwise and nine times counterclockwise

FIGURE 3-51

Tilt T–11

T–11 and up. As you continue to practice in this way, the whole procedure will take less and less time until it finally becomes simply moments.

c. Inhale and pull the CHI from the T–11 up to C–7. (Figure 3–52) Push from the sternum to tilt the C–7 back. Tuck in the chin, clench the teeth (Figure 3–53(a)), squeeze the temples (Figure 3–53(b)) and the occipital bone, and press the tongue firmly to the roof of the mouth. (Figure 3–53(c)) This will create a tension similar to the tension of the arched bow discussed previously which is now ready to

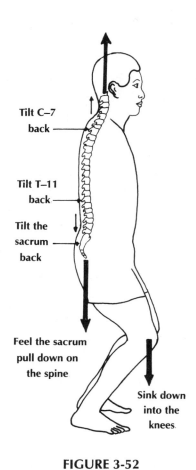

Tilt C–7 back

Tilt T–11 back

Tilt the sacrum back

Feel the sacrum pull down on the spine

Sink down into the knees.

FIGURE 3-52

Pull the CHI from T–11 up to C–7

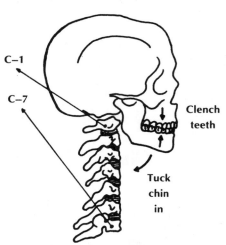

C–1

C–7

Clench teeth

Tuck chin in

(a) Clench the teeth. Sink the chin in

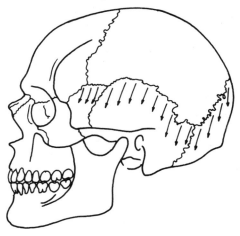

(b) Squeeze the temple bones

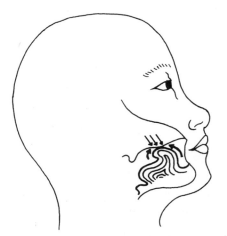

(c) Press the tongue firmly to the roof of the mouth

FIGURE 3-53

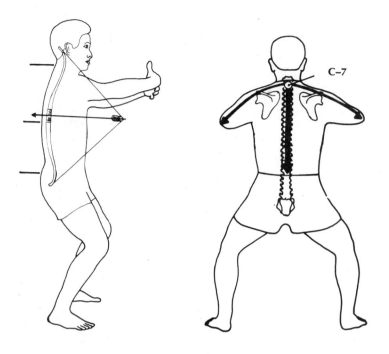

(a) Create a tension similar
to a fully arched bow

(b) As you push from the sternum to C–7,
the spine and shoulders will connect

FIGURE 3-54

release an arrow. (Figure 3–54(a)) The whole neck will be connected to the spine and sacrum, and to the legs and heels. (Figure 3-54(b)) As the energy moves up from the sacrum to C–7, the major push of internal force occurs. (C–7, T–11 and the sacrum are known as the "stations of internal force".) Once you can develop and feel the force in the C–7, you will be able to exert the force. This entire process is called self-adjustment of the cranial pump and will activate the cranial

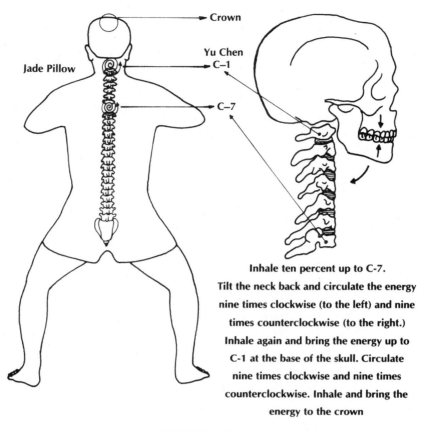

Jade Pillow

Crown

Yu Chen
C–1

C–7

Inhale ten percent up to C-7.
Tilt the neck back and circulate the energy
nine times clockwise (to the left) and nine
times counterclockwise (to the right.)
Inhale again and bring the energy up to
C-1 at the base of the skull. Circulate
nine times clockwise and nine times
counterclockwise. Inhale and bring the
energy to the crown

FIGURE 3-55

Self-Adjustment of the Cranial Pump

pump. (Figure 3-55) The action of the cranial pump will greatly increase, thereby increasing brain power as well. Circle nine times clockwise and nine times counterclockwise at C–7. Feel the CHI energy join the scapulae, the arms, and the hands and fingers together. You will feel the CHI start to flow from the thumb and fingers of one hand to the thumb and fingers of the other hand, like a jumper cable. Use the eyes to look at the thumbs and direct the CHI to that point.

d. If you are out of breath or cannot go on, exhale a little bit and then inhale again. If you cannot do this, you can simply exhale and bring the CHI up to the crown, omitting the Yu Chen (Jade Pillow, BL–9 or Base of the Skull). If you can continue, bring the CHI up to the Yu-Chen and circle it nine times both clockwise and counterclockwise as you did at the points previously described, until you feel that CHI has developed there. (Figure 3-55)

e. Inhale and pull the CHI up to the crown (Figure 3–55), the seat of the pineal gland located at the top of the head, by looking up with your eyes. (Figure 3–56(a)) Concentrate on the Pai Hui at the crown and circle it again nine times clockwise and nine times counterclockwise, using your mind and your eyes, until energy is experienced there. (Figure 3–56(b)) Feel the energy flow from the sacrum to the Door of Life, to T–11, to C–7, to the occipital bone, and to the crown as they become fused into one channel and linked together. If you are out of breath, you can pull up and exhale. Normalize your breathing.

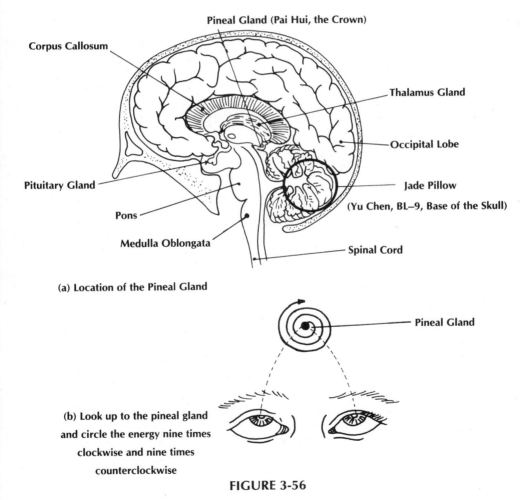

(a) Location of the Pineal Gland

(b) Look up to the pineal gland and circle the energy nine times clockwise and nine times counterclockwise

FIGURE 3-56

Circle the energy in the pineal gland

137

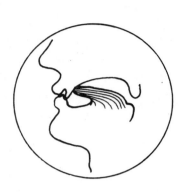

(a) The tongue is on the roof of the mouth

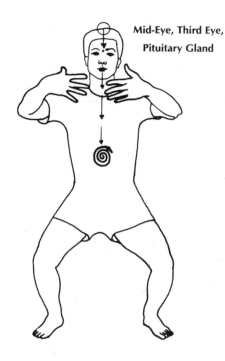

Mid-Eye, Third Eye,
Pituitary Gland

(b) Bring the energy down to the third eye

(c) Bring the energy down to the solar plexus

FIGURE 3-57

f. Make sure that the tongue is up on the roof of the mouth. (Figure 3–57(a)) Bring the energy down to the mid-eye, concentrating there for a while while practicing normalized breathing, until you feel the energy build up. (Figure 3–57(b)) Then bring the energy down to the palate where the tongue will serve as a switch joining the Governor Channel to the Functional Channel. Bring the CHI down to the throat, heart center and solar plexus (Chung Wan, CO–12), circling it nine times in both directions, until you feel energy enlivened there again. (Figure 3–57(c)) Use the eyes to help in this circulation.

g. Finally, bring the energy to the navel. (Figure 3–58(a)) Concentrate there until you feel CHI freely go down to it. Listen and look inside. Feel the sensation of the flow of CHI in one circulating motion from the navel to the perineum, to the soles, up to the knees, to the perineum again, and up to the sacrum, to the spine, to the crown and down to the third eye, to the throat, to the heart and to the navel. (Figure 3–58(b)) When you feel the circle is moving well, simply let it flow by itself. Feel the navel warm and fill with CHI.

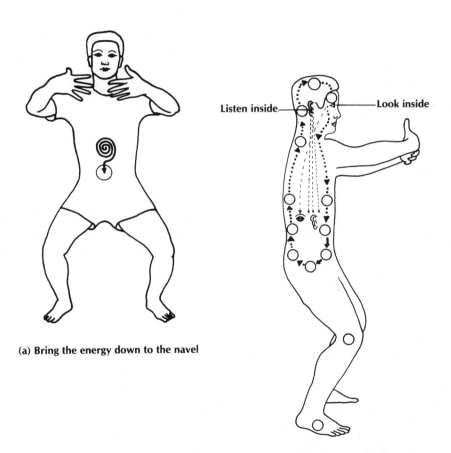

(a) Bring the energy down to the navel

Listen inside ——— Look inside

(b) Feel the sensation of the flow of CHI

FIGURE 3-58

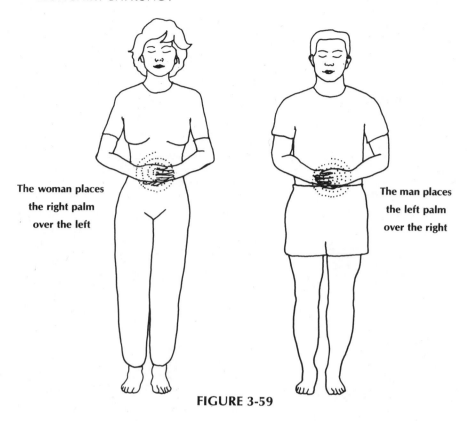

The woman places the right palm over the left

The man places the left palm over the right

FIGURE 3-59

Stand up straight and put the palms over the navel

Remember as you complete the final stage to stand still and relax all of the body's muscles, holding this position for as long as possible. Simply standing and experiencing this powerful energy flow for ten to fifteen minutes will shorten the time necessary to master the Iron Shirt techniques by as much as one to three hours. You have created a tremendous CHI pressure and your mind will condense and direct the flow. Feel the energy flow in the Microcosmic Orbit.

Stand up straight, continue to touch the tongue to the palate, and put the palms over the navel. Men put the right palm over the navel, covering it with the left palm. Women put the left palm over the navel, covering it with the right palm. (Figure 3–59) Concentrate on the navel for a while, feeling the energy that is generated by the Chi Kung. As you are standing, practice the Bone Breathing Process described below.

10. Bone Breathing Process

a. The Bone Breathing Process is practiced immediately after you finish the First Stage, the Second Stage and finally, after the Third, and final, Stage of this exercise, to bring the energy down to the navel. At this time, your body is still filled with energy. To practice the Bone Breathing Process you can use Embracing the Tree or any position that you are in at the time.

Bone Breathing or bone compression is the method of "Cleansing the Marrow", or cleaning out fat in the bone marrow so that you can direct and absorb the creative (sexual) energy into the bone to help regrow the bone marrow. (Figure 3–60) During this process, we take advantage of the CHI generated in Iron Shirt I by absorbing CHI into the bones, thereby greatly increasing the circulation of CHI. With in-

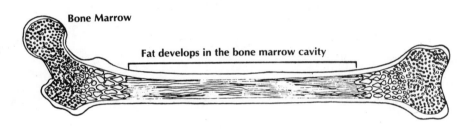

Bone Marrow

Fat develops in the bone marrow cavity

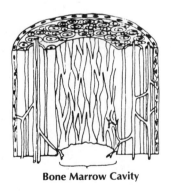

Bone Marrow Cavity

FIGURE 3-60

Bone Marrow

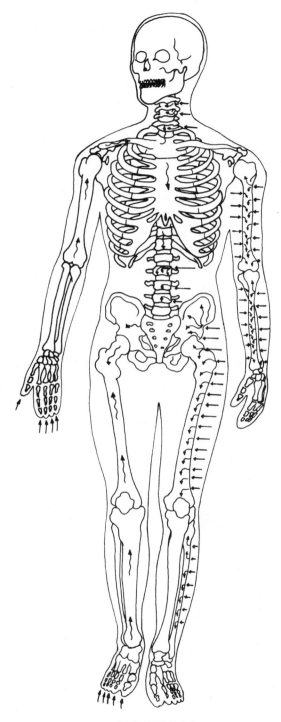

FIGURE 3-61

Use the mind and eye power to breathe CHI through the fingertips and toes, up
the arms and legs, and up the spinal column to the skull

creased circulation, the CHI is permitted to flow freely into the bones and the blood, carrying necessary nutrients and oxygen, and is permitted to circulate freely throughout the body. Tension in the muscles surrounding the bones is lessened. The bones become strong and healthy because the marrow, as the major product of red and white blood cells, now has room to grow.

This process takes time to practice. It is most important that you relax and are not tense when you practice Bone Breathing.

Bone Breathing is a two stage process:

(1) Inhale and exhale as though through the fingers and toes: In the first stage of the Bone Breathing Process, by using the powers of the mind and the eyes, outside energy is breathed in through the fingertips and toes, gradually up to the hands and arms to the skull, and then down the spinal column and legs. (Figure 3–61) A sensation is felt as you breathe into each area. Some people report a numbness, others a fullness, still others a tingling, or "something different" in their bones. Many people claim to feel more in their legs. When you inhale through the fingers, the feeling is cool. When you exhale, the feeling is warm. Feel inside the bones. No matter what you feel, Bone Breathing is practiced to cleanse the fat stored in the bone marrow to make room for positive energy, such as creative energy (sexual power), which will allow the bones to store, rebuild and grow the marrow.

(2) Inhale and exhale the same way through the toes: In the second stage, inhale through the toes and then, by degrees, inhale up to and into the thigh bones. After inhaling, hold your breath, but not so long that you experience discomfort. Then, exhale down and out through the toes. In the next progression, inhale up through the legs and into the hips, then exhale down and out through the legs. When you have accomplished this, breathe in through the legs to the sacrum. Here, you may feel energy surge up through the back and throughout the entire nervous system. Breathe up the back; the breath will be quite long at this point.

Finally, while you breathe through the legs and up the back, also breathe in through the fingers, up into the arms and shoulders, through C–7 and into the head.

Keep in mind that energy is absorbed and ejected more effectively at appointed places such as the toes, fingertips, elbows, knees, sacrum, C–7, Door of Life, shoulders, or tip of the nose. (Figure 3–62)

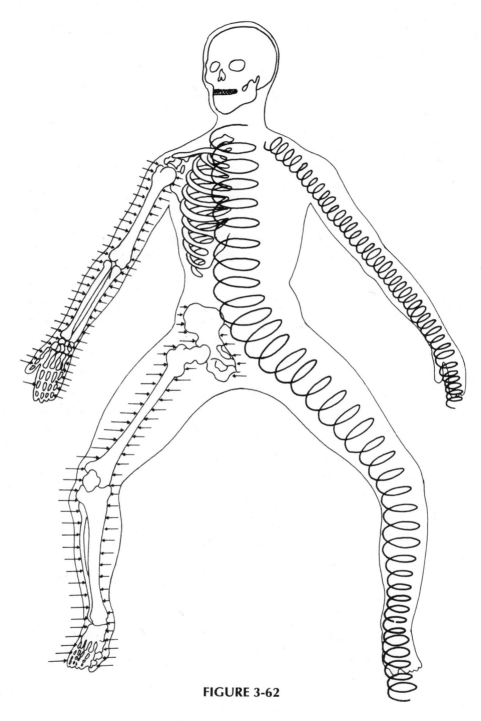

FIGURE 3-62

In advanced techniques, you will learn to breathe through the skin to push the
CHI into the bones and wrap the CHI around the bones

11. Power Exercise

a. This exercise is another means of increasing the flow of CHI to the bones, squeezing out the toxins, sediment and waste materials, as well as the negative emotions that have become stored in the muscles.

(1) Muscles and the Emotions Stored within Them

In this stressful life, pollution and chemicals accumulate in the system, depositing in our organs. In the Tao System we believe that all negative and positive emotions are also stored in the organs. When the organs are filled with toxins, sediment, waste materials and too many negative emotions, these substances will back up into the muscle which handles the overflow of each organ, similar to a backup tank. If we do not squeeze the muscles by increasing the flow of CHI, thereby eliminating the undesirable elements and emotions which have been stored there, the muscles will be very tense and clamp onto the bones. As a result, the person will constantly have the feeling of stress.

Once the negative emotions are cleaned out, the positive emotions have more room to grow. Positive emotions make the muscles relaxed and loose. The explanation below gives details of muscles and the emotions that become stored there. This information is contributed by Larry Short, the founder of the institute for Total Person Facilitation (T.P.F.).

Muscles and Their Associated Negative/Positive Emotions

Hands
- − Fear of losing grip
- + Belonging, reaching out

Forearms

Brachioradialis and forearm extensors/flexors

Correspond to Stomach—appropriate meridians
- − Rejection
- − Fear of attack
- + Acceptance
- + Recognizing the way to proceed

Upper arms

Correspond to Stomach and Spleen

Biceps and Triceps, Deltoids

Correspond to Lungs
- − I can't do it
- − Weakness, fear of lack of capacity
- − Sorrow, loss
- + I can do it
- + Strength
- + Responsibility

Scapulae
Correspond to Triple Heater
  − Fear of taking risks; not willing
    to take risks
  − Cowardly
  + Vitality, radiant power, life-
    force, responsive action
  + Brave
SCM, Scaleanus, and Neck
  Muscles
Correspond to Stomach
Upper Trapezius Muscles
Correspond to Kidneys
  − Guilt
  − Fear, turtle hiding
  + Responsive
  + Expressive
  + Taking risks
Feet
Correspond to Spine
  − Insecurity
  + Taking a stand, projects, leav-
    ing your mark in the world
Lower legs, Calves
Correspond to Adrenals and
  Triple Heater
Gastrocremias
Soleus
  − Hesitation, fear of going for-
    ward, waiting
  + Setting the stage, preparing
Upper legs, Quadriceps
Correspond to Small Intestines
  − Lack of support
  + Feeling supported
Hips, Psoas/Iliacus
Correspond to Kidneys

  − Fear Gluteus (Muscles of But-
    tocks)
  − Disloyalty, lack of commitment
  + Loyalty, commitment, letting go
Sacrum, Piriformis
Correspond to Circulation/sex
  − Insecurity
  + Security, rootedness, grounded,
    stable
Lumbar spine, Sacrospinalis
Correspond to Bladder
  − Fear of being taken advantage
    of and/or of being cheated
  + Ability, bravery, courage, ability
    to take charge of situation
Thoracic spine and rib cage,
  Spine
Correspond to Bladder
  − Fear, cowardice, running away
  + Ability to perform
Ribs
Correspond to Lungs
  − Sorrow and grief
  + Vitality, surrender, openness
Cervical spine
  Corresponds to Neck extensors
  − Inappropriateness, tiredness
  + Clarity
Skull
Corresponds to Breathing
Head
Corresponds to Temple
  − Dullness, confusion, distraction
  + Environmental awareness,
    being present, being here and
    now

Jaw, Masseter, Pterygoids
Correspond to Stomach
 − Frustration
 + Knowing what you want and
   need

Occiput
Corresponds to Back of skull

 + Inspiration
 − Dullness, worry

Sternum, Pectoralis muscles
Correspond to Liver
 − Anger, resentment
 + Openness, valiance, dignity

The Power Exercise, also known as Dynamic Tension, will greatly tone up the body muscles by simply a few minutes practice each day instead of an hour of workouts. (Figure 3–63) In this exercise you

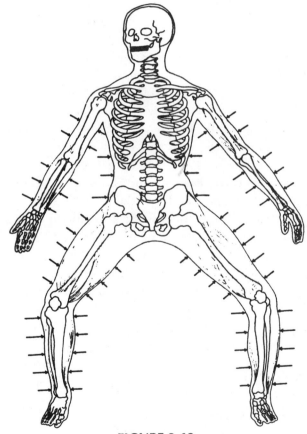

FIGURE 3-63

**Dynamic tension tones up the body muscles, permitting compression of muscles
and bones**

evenly work out every muscle and will not overtire them. Studies of the proper tension of these muscles for a few minutes each day have been made which indicate that these exercises develop good muscle tone.

If you tire in the standing position, rest and walk for a while and then resume the same position practiced in Embracing the Tree, or you can simply continue from the Bone Breathing Process.

(1) Relax the hand muscles. Then, use the mind to tighten the hand muscles and squeeze the muscles to the bones of the radius and ulna (the bones of the forearm) tightly. Hold the muscles firmly to the bones for 30 to 60 seconds. Exhale strongly through the mouth, then totally relax the muscles and the shoulders. Feel the rush of CHI as the toxic tensions and negative emotions, such as fear of attack, leave the muscles. Feel the positive emotions, such as recognizing the way to proceed, letting the life-force enter into the muscles.

(2) Relax the arm muscles. Inhale and spread the arm muscles into the humerus (the bone of the upper arm). Tighten the muscles all around the arm. Hold them tightly for 30 to 60 seconds. Exhale and release them. Let go of the fear that you cannot do it. Let go of weakness. Release the feelings of sorrow and loss. Let positive emotions enter into these muscles. Feel that you can do it. Feel that you are strong, and that you have capacity and can take on responsibility.

(3) Relax the legs. Inhale and squeeze the muscles around the fibula and tibia (the bones of the lower leg) tightly to the bones. Hold them tightly for 30 to 60 seconds and exhale. Relax the muscles, letting go of the toxins and accumulated negative emotions such as hesitation and procrastination. Allow the positive emotions to enter such as preparedness or readiness to grow. Be totally aware of the CHI that is generated.

(4) Relax the thighs. Inhale and squeeze the muscles around the femur (the bone of the upper leg) tightly to the bones and hold for 30 to 60 seconds. Exhale and relax the muscles away from the bones. Release the feeling of lack of support; let the feeling of support grow. Be aware of the CHI flowing between the bone and muscle.

(5) Relax the neck. Inhale and squeeze the neck, the head muscles and the cervical (the neck) muscles tightly, holding the squeeze for 30 to 60 seconds. Relax and let go of guilt and fear. Feel the positive

growth of expressiveness, responsiveness and taking risks.

(6) Relax the back, especially the spinal cord, and the chest. Inhale and tightly squeeze the muscles around the spinal cord from the Thoracic vertebrae, down to the lumbar vertebrae to the sacrum as well as the rib cage of the chest. Hold for 30 to 60 seconds. Release the entire spinal cord and the rib cage. Relax and let go of the fear of being taken advantage of or being cheated. Eliminate cowardice and the desire to run away. Release sorrow, grief and tiredness. Grow the positive feelings of bravery, openness and the ability to take charge and to perform.

(7) After you have practiced well for one to two weeks, you can do exercises (1) through (6) all at once by starting from the hands to the legs, to the neck and head, to the spinal cord and rib cage. Hold the squeeze for 30 to 60 seconds and release totally. Feel the muscles and bones separate from each other.

(8) When you finish the exercise, stand up straight and put the palm on the navel. Men should put the right hand on the navel, covered with the left palm. Women should place the left hand on the navel with the right palm over it. Stand still for a while and feel how the CHI flows. Then, concentrate on collecting the energy into the navel. In the beginning, you can use the hand to assist in the collection of energy.

(a) Men, starting at the navel, should spiral the energy out in a clockwise direction, making 36 revolutions, being careful not to go above the diaphram or below the pubic bone. Circling out beyond the pubic bone allows the energy to leak out. Once you have completed the clockwise revolutions, spiral inwards in the opposite direction 24 times, ending and collecting the energy at the navel.

(b) Women should do the same thing, but begin by spiraling the energy out from the navel in a counterclockwise direction, and spiraling back to the navel in a clockwise direction.

Spend one to two weeks on this practice. Review the Microcosmic Orbit Meditation for circulation of the CHI in Chapter 2 of this book.

When you become proficient at using the mind in this practice, you need only use the mind to circulate the CHI.

When you are finished, walk. If you feel the chest tighten or any congestion, use the palms and gently brush down the chest to bring the CHI down.

(c) Once you have completed the circuit, you will need less time to practice it in preparation for this Embracing The Tree stance. Thereafter, raise the energy up to your head to the Pai Hui (Crown). Once the energy arrives there, you should feel as though something were pushing up through the crown of the head. Always end by returning the energy to the navel.

B. Embracing the Tree Stance (Practical Procedure)

1. The Exercise (Figure 3–64)

When you have practiced well and understand each part of the previous exercises, you can proceed with the next practice as described below.

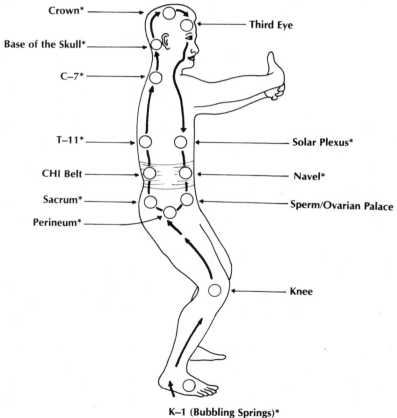

FIGURE 3-64

Embracing the Tree

*Circle the energy nine times clockwise and nine times counterclockwise

a. Assume a Horse Stance. Sink down onto the hips, keeping the back straight and holding the legs apart in the standard length of the lower legs. Turn the toes inward so that the feet are positioned as though on the circumference of a circle. The knees are well bent and the groin area is relaxed and open.

b. Extend the arms out in front of you at shoulder height as though you were encircling the trunk of a tree. The palms face you. The fingers are gently separated with the thumbs pointing up and the fingertips are held apart a distance of about the width of the face. Feel as though you were lightly holding a ball between your hands.

c. Place the tongue on the palate. Breathe in and out deeply nine to eighteen times so that each time that you exhale, the abdomen contracts and the thoracic diaphragm goes up into the chest, compressing the lungs and pulling the sexual organs up. When you inhale, the thoracic diaphragm goes down to compress the abdomen so that you can feel the perineum bulge outward.

d. After you have exhaled for the ninth, eighteenth or 36th time, inhale ten percent of your total capacity to the level of the navel, while keeping the abdomen flat. Pull up the sexual organs, or close the vagina tight, and pull the anus closed. Inhale again and pull up the left and right anus, bringing CHI to the kidneys. Wrap and pack the CHI in the kidneys, then circle the energy in the navel nine times clockwise and nine times counterclockwise to collect the energy there, pausing until you feel the need to breath again.

e. Inhale ten percent of your capacity down to three inches below the navel or, for women, the Ovary Palace. Pack the CHI in this region. Inhale down to the lower abdominal area or, for men, the Sperm Palace and hold it again until you feel the need to breathe. Inhale ten percent more of your capacity down to the perineum and hold it as long as you comfortably can. You can keep on inhaling and packing in as long as you feel comfortable. Sometimes you can exhale a little bit so that you can inhale more. In the beginning, start by inhaling less air in a short period of time. When you are well-trained, you can hold more air for a longer time.

f. Exhale and send energy down the backs of the legs into the ground. The feet will fill with the energy and you should feel the palms and soles "breathing". Breathe through the palms and soles. Regulate your breath.

151

g. Apply pressure, especially with the big toes. Feel that you are "sucking" energy up out of the earth through the "Bubbling Springs" in the soles of the feet (K–1 point). "Claw" the floor with the feet. Inhale and draw the energy out of the ground. Collect energy there by circling the sole (K–1) with energy nine times clockwise and nine times counterclockwise. Contract the muscles of the anus and groin and pull up the testicles or vagina and anus. Bring the energy up the front of the legs to the knees, hold the CHI at the knees and lock the knees by turning them slightly outward. Bring the energy to the buttocks by curving in the upper thigh and then bring the energy into the perineum. Hold the CHI here and circle it nine times clockwise and nine times counterclockwise. Exhale and regulate the breath by Energizer Breathing nine to eighteen times and continue to feel the palms and soles breathe.

h. Inhale ten percent, pulling up the left and right anus and packing the back area and kidneys.

i. Contract the back part of the anus to bring CHI up to the sacrum. Pull up the testicles or vagina. Put pressure on the sacrum and tuck it back, but do not tilt the hips. This pushes the lower back (lumbar vertebrae) out and straightens curves in the spine. Inhale ten percent of your capacity and pack CHI into the sacrum. Collect the energy there by mentally circling it nine times clockwise and nine times counterclockwise. Continue to contract the anus.

j. Inhale ten percent of your capacity again. Pull the CHI up to T–11 and tilt the back to a straight position. Collect the energy there by circling nine times clockwise and counterclockwise within a three inch area.

k. Inhale ten percent of your capacity and pack more at the whole back. Continue to tighten the anus and groin, pull up the testicles or squeeze the vagina, tighten the neck, sink the sternum, and push from the sternum to tilt C–7 back.

l. Tuck the chin in to lock the neck, keeping the chest relaxed. With this action, the energy moves from the sacrum to C–7. Pack the CHI at C–7 by circling the energy nine times clockwise and nine times counterclockwise. This will activate the cranial pump located at the base of the skull (the Jade Pillow, C–1) which works in tandem with the sacral pump to move cerebrospinal fluid up the back. The sacral and cranial pumps activate the cerebrospinal fluid in the spine and brain.

m. With your neck still tight, inhale, packing energy up to your Jade Pillow. Collect it, circling nine times clockwise and nine times counterclockwise.

n. Inhale ten percent and pull up to the crown of the head. Stop, turn both eyes up, and look inward to the area of the pineal gland, circling nine times clockwise and nine times counterclockwise, until you are out of breath. Exhale slowly. Relax the neck, anus, groin and urogenital diaphragm. Keep the tongue at the palate.

o. Regulate the breath by Energizer Breathing, but exhale more and inhale less. Concentrate on the third eye. Guide the energy down from the tongue past the throat, heart center and down to the solar plexus. Collect the CHI in the solar plexus, circling nine times clockwise and nine times counterclockwise.

p. With the toes extended, open the knees slightly so that you can feel the force in the ankle joints. This will enable you to grasp the ground with the feet, and feel the soles press down to the ground. Force the energy to flow down inside, putting the dynamic tension on the small and big balls of the feet and to the outer edges, like axles running from the outside of the ankles to the big toes. Make sure you do not lift any of the feet's nine points of contact off the ground.

q. Stand still, maintaining the position. Feel the energy travel out of the ground, up the legs and into the spinal cord, through C-7 at the base of the neck out into the arms, up to the pineal and pituitary glands, and then down the front of the body to the navel. Feel heat in the navel and continue circulating the energy for as long as you wish.

r. Practice the Bone Breathing Process.

s. Practice the Power Exercise.

t. Stand erect, keep the tongue at the palate, and collect energy in the navel. (Figure 3–65)

u. Walk slowly and breathe normally. Stroke the chest downward with the palms of the hands to prevent or counteract any congestion that might develop there and walk about to distribute CHI and give the stressed muscles a chance to recuperate. (Figure 3–66)

Keep the abdomen soft. Remember that softness makes energy: it is said that soft makes strong. To achieve this, keep the muscles in a soft tension.

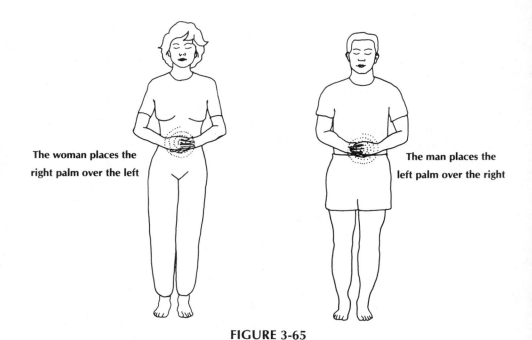

The woman places the right palm over the left

The man places the left palm over the right

FIGURE 3-65

Place the palms over the navel to collect the energy

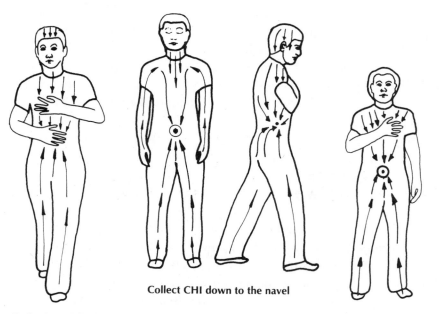

Walk slowly and stroke the chest

Collect CHI down to the navel

Stroke the chest downward with the palms

FIGURE 3-66

In time, you should be able to do Embracing the Tree in two breaths: one down the front and one up the back. With practice, if you are relaxed, you can do the whole process in just one breath. The stance strengthens the muscle-tendon lines (meridians) that travel through the thumbs and big toes.

You may have already discovered that all Iron Shirt work exercises the body and instills confidence.

C. Summary of Embracing the Tree (Figure 3–67)

1. Stand with the feet a knee-to-toe length apart; press the sacrum down; round the scapulae; relax the chest; hold the head erect; po-

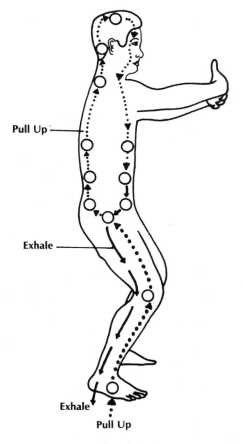

Pull Up

Exhale

Exhale

Pull Up

FIGURE 3-67

Circulating the energy during Embracing the Tree

sition the arms as if they were encircling a tree; hold the thumbs up; relax the fingers, barely permitting them to touch.

2. Practice lower abdominal breathing nine to eighteen times. When you do abdominal breathing, emphasize inhalation by rounding the abdomen and exhalation by flattening the abdomen on all sides. Feel the sexual organs move up and down with the breath.

3. Exhale; flatten the stomach; lower the diaphragm.

4. Inhale, tightening the perineum and anus by pulling up the middle anus, then the left and right sides of the anus. Feel the CHI energy go up to both kidneys and pack into them. Pull up the sexual organs. (Remember that the anal muscle has a close relationship with all organs and glands.) Pack into the navel without expanding the abdomen. Keep the chest relaxed and the abdomen soft, and spiral first nine times clockwise, then nine times counterclockwise, making a circle of about one and one-half inches in radius.

5. Breathe into the middle abdomen, without spiraling, and pack.

6. Breathe into the lower abdomen, without spiraling.

7. Breathe into the perineum and feel it bulge out.

8. Exhale through the legs and feet down to about six inches into the ground. Feel the palms and soles breathing and use the lower abdominal breathing.

9. Inhale, tighten the perineum, and press the soles of the feet into the ground. Claw the toes and spiral at the kidney points (K–1) on the soles, nine times clockwise and nine times counterclockwise, both spirals moving simultaneously in the same direction.

10. Inhale, bringing energy to the knees. Lock the knees, without spiraling.

11. Inhale up to the perineum, and spiral nine times clockwise and nine times counterclockwise. Feel the bulge.

12. Exhale. Regulate the breath, and be aware of the soles and palms breathing.

13. Inhale up to the sacrum, tilt the sacrum back, packing it, and spiral nine times clockwise and nine times counterclockwise. This will strengthen and activate the sacral pump.

14. Inhale to T–11, inflating the kidney area, and press out on the lower back to straighten the curve there, spiraling nine times clockwise and nine times counterclockwise.

15. Inhale to C–7, straightening the curve at the neck, and lock the

neck. Spiral nine times clockwise and nine times counterclockwise.

16. Inhale to the Jade Pillow, clench the teeth tight, and squeeze the skull and the temple bones to strengthen and activate the cranial pump. Spiral nine times clockwise and nine times counterclockwise.

17. Inhale to the crown (pineal gland) and spiral nine times clockwise and nine times counterclockwise. If you cannot go all the way up on one breath, you can pass over the Jade Pillow or take an extra breath where needed until your capacity increases.

18. Exhale with the tongue up to the palate. Regulate the breath.

19. Concentrate on the third eye, until you feel the CHI build up there. Bring the energy down to the solar plexus and spiral nine times clockwise and nine times counterclockwise. Bring the CHI down to the navel. Stand still and maintain this position.

20. Stand up and bring the energy into the navel, putting your hands over the navel and bringing the feet together. Relax. Collect the energy in the navel area. When you feel calm, walk around and brush the energy down, if necessary.

21. Practice the Bone Breathing Process.

22. Practice the Power Exercise.

III. ROOTING, COLLECTING CHI ENERGY, ILLUSTRATIONS OF POSTURES

A. Rooting Practice

The Rooting Practice is very important in the Healing Tao System. Rooting can be compared to the foundation of a building. The stronger the foundation, the higher the building may be built, and the more difficult it is to topple.

After mastering the Rooting Practice you will feel, as you walk around, stand, or sit in your daily life, that you are more in touch with the earth. (Figure 3–68) You will feel more stable and practical minded, not "spacey". Many Healing Tao students, after practicing Iron Shirt Rooting for a while, find that they have good balance and greatly improve the quality of their physical activities, such as running, skiing, tennis and Yoga.

Taoist Practitioners are very concerned with rootedness. The more

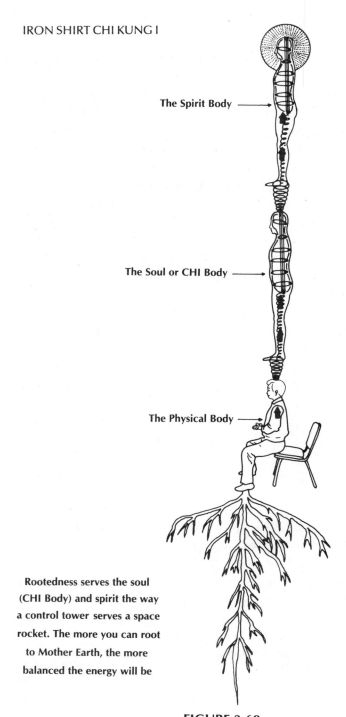

The Spirit Body

The Soul or CHI Body

The Physical Body

Rootedness serves the soul
(CHI Body) and spirit the way
a control tower serves a space
rocket. The more you can root
to Mother Earth, the more
balanced the energy will be

FIGURE 3-68

Rootedness to Mother Earth

he or she can root to Mother Earth, the more balanced the energy will be. Such a balance of energy increases healing energy. In advanced practice, rooting is required to perform the practice of the Thrusting Channels and Belt Channels. Tai Chi, the Healing Hand and the higher spiritual practices draw upon the earth energy, as well as heavenly energy, to transform life-force energy into spiritual energy in order to give birth to the soul and spirit. It is the earth energy which helps the soul and spirit grow. Astral traveling requires rooting, and this earthly rootedness serves the soul and spirit the way a control tower serves a space rocket. Those who try to bring CHI up to the head, or receive heavenly energy without grounding in the earth, become "spacey" instead of "in tune" with their experience.

Always balance out by using both sides of the body during practice.

Developing the Rooting Practice requires two people: one to push and the other to stand. This exercise will greatly improve your stance. Many people will find that one side is weaker than the other, or the upper part, such as the neck, is weaker than the lower part. Practice on the strong side first and then the weak side so that you will have a reference for improving the weak side.

Gradually you will grow stronger and it will require less effort to maintain your structured position because you will have built extra muscles and strengthened the tendons, tendon attachment sites and fasciae as one structure. When you "root" properly, it feels as if you are sucking the ground, or have grown a deep root into the earth. This is because the whole structure, as a unit, is pressing into the ground. You can feel the entire bone structure sink down to the ground.

With practice you will be able to bring energy along the prescribed course more quickly and easily. To test your rootedness, find a partner who can push you while you hold the structure.

1. The Stance

The purpose of the Iron Shirt Rooting Principle is to line up the bone structure with the joints to feel the whole body become one piece. Once you become proficient in the practice, you will position yourself in the proper structure quite easily. Stand in the Iron Shirt

Horse Stance. Sometimes you can stand with the feet at a slightly wider position. However, if the feet are too wide apart, you have to use muscle strength to hold the whole body together. When the force comes, the muscle will hold the force and knock the alignment off. If the position of the feet is too narrow, you will be using the tendons' force to help hold the structure together, affecting alignment as well.

When your partner pushes you with force, your neck must be relaxed so that the force will not go into the neck, causing pain there. Your structure, inner organs, and tendons, muscles and fasciae must work as a whole to hold the position. This will gradually increase your inner strength.

2. The CHI Belt

Packing CHI into the organs is very important in the practice of rooting. It is particularly important to pack CHI in the kidneys and to join the kidneys and K–1 (Bubbling Springs) into one line. The navel and the two kidneys must join together feeling like a large belt, belted across your waist. (Figure 3-69(a)) The joining of the navel, the sides of the waist, the two kidneys and T–11 with CHI energy is basic to the rooting principle and is called the "CHI Belt".

Without the CHI Belt, the major connection of the upper and lower energy joints, the structure and CHI will be lost. To develop the CHI Belt, first pack CHI in the kidneys and the navel, expanding first from the left kidney out to the left waist, then towards the front to the navel. Expand, pack and wrap the right kidney to the right waist, and then forward to the navel. This joins both sides together at the navel. As the CHI Belt expands, it connects to the T–11 and the Door of Life. The navel now feels like a full blown tire encased within a big belt. Once you experience a CHI Belt in the rooting practice, you will be able to attain rootedness quickly and will not need to use your muscles to join your structure together. Therefore, mastering the CHI Belt will help you to be very relaxed in your practice.

3. The Principle of Rooting

    a. Assume Embracing the Tree.
    b. Sink the energy down to the lower navel area.

c. Sink down as comfortably as you can, and open the groin by slightly separating the knees.

d. The toes turn slightly inward. When the knee caps are locked (meaning that the knee joints are held tightly), the knees will lock in the ankle joints like the position assumed when you are sitting astride a saddle. Sink into the knees. You can feel the connection between the knees and the ankle joints and the connection down to the feet. Feel your whole body weight drop down to the ground. The force passes through the bone structure. (Figure 3–69(b)) Feel the bones like sponges that absorb the force and direct it to the ground.

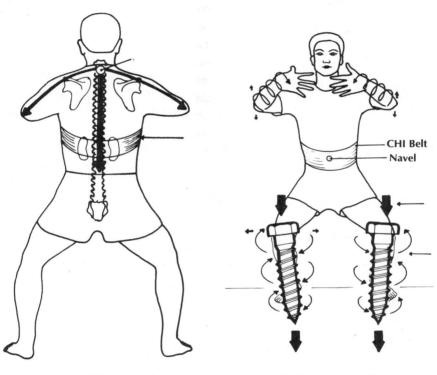

CHI Belt
Navel

(a) The Chi Belt joins the whole body structure together

(b) Press down and turn the knee outwards to screw the force into the ground

FIGURE 3-69

The Principles of Rooting

e. The hands are at shoulder level, the elbows sink. Feel the force of the sinking elbows pressing into the bone structure. If the elbows are up, you will disconnect from the tendon power.

f. Line up the shoulders, joining the scapulae with the spine by rounding the scapulae and sinking the chest. Connect through the hip joints down to the knee and ankle joints.

Line up the shoulder joints by pushing the thumbs out and the pinky fingers in, feeling the tendons pull. The wrist joints are connected to the shoulders. Relax the neck, especially the trapezius muscle, so that the connection does not go up to the head which will bring force to the neck. Otherwise, when your partner pushes you, you will feel like you were hit by a two-by-four, and it will knock you over. When you relax the neck and join the shoulders with the spine, the force travels down the spine and down to the ground.

To connect the shoulder joints with the spine, you need to round the scapulae and sink the chest so that the force can be transferred from the shoulders to the scapulae. Then, push the neck straight and the T–11 out. Keep the sacrum straight without moving the hips, until you feel the spine as a flexed bow, full of strength. All becomes one line. When the groin area is open, the hip joints will join with the knees, the feet, and all will join down with the ground. Feel the CHI Belt, belting the waist and joining the entire structure together.

4. The Practice of Rooting

Having a partner push against you can increase your rooting power and thus strengthen the fasciae and spinal cord, increasing the function of the sacrum and cranial pump.

Assume the position for Embracing The Tree, and pack with air as described. Your partner should then push (not hit) his fist against your sacrum, T–11, C-7, and the base of the skull, respectively. It is important that these four centers become strengthened and linked together into one line. If they are not linked, they become many unconnected lines, and the partner's force will not travel down to the ground properly.

The spinal cord is the house of the nervous system which joins all the other parts of the body. The spine consists of many bones which are put together and held by muscles, tendons and fasciae. Most of the exercises are not to strengthen the spine solely. However, Iron Shirt Chi Kung is designed to strengthen the entire bone structure, especially the spine. Many people have weak spines which cause bad posture, breathing problems and weak organs. Weak organs are the original cause of a weak spine. Poor posture becomes a vicious cycle: organs are kept weak because CHI cannot circulate throughout the various body systems. Iron Shirt (1) protects organs which generate vital CHI; (2) recharges them with packing; (3) circulates CHI up the spine and strengthens the nervous system; and (4) creates the storage space for the CHI energy by burning out fat.

5. Strengthening the Sacral Pump (Figure 3–70)

The sacrum is the very important pump that moves CHI into the spine. Assume the Embracing the Tree stance. Be aware of your sacrum, pack with CHI, develop a CHI Belt, and have your partner put his fist right on the sacrum. Slowly tilt the sacrum to the back, pushing against your partner's hand, with very little movement from the hip. Have your partner push you as much as you can withstand without being pushed over, and gradually increase the push until you grow more powerful in the sacrum area. Hold this position for one to two minutes. Breathe normally.

Be aware of the force of your partner being transferred from your sacrum to the legs, to the feet and to the toes. You can exert force from the toes back up the feet to the heels, to the legs and to the sacrum.

When your partner releases you, rest for a while and feel that the sacrum is open and feel how the CHI flows up the spine.

When you are advanced in the practice, you can be very relaxed. There is no need to pack. Simply feel the force pass from the sacrum to the ground, and feel the ground force come up to resist the force through use of the bones. Do not lean towards your partner.

6. Strengthening T–11

T–11, or the eleventh Thoracic Vertebra (the point of the adrenal gland and the kidneys), is regarded by the Taoist as a pump which

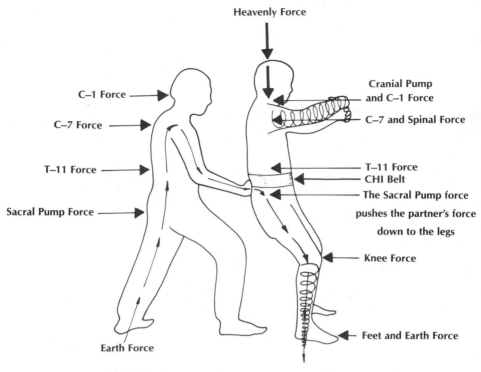

Heavenly Force

C–1 Force

C–7 Force

T–11 Force

Sacral Pump Force

Earth Force

Cranial Pump and C–1 Force

C–7 and Spinal Force

T–11 Force

CHI Belt

The Sacral Pump force pushes the partner's force down to the legs

Knee Force

Feet and Earth Force

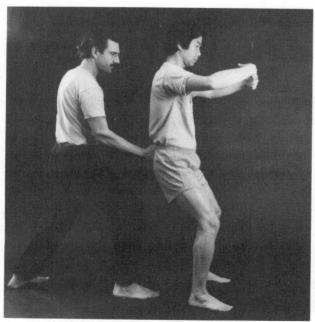

FIGURE 3-70

The partner's force is transferred down to the ground through the bone
structure by the force of the sacral pump

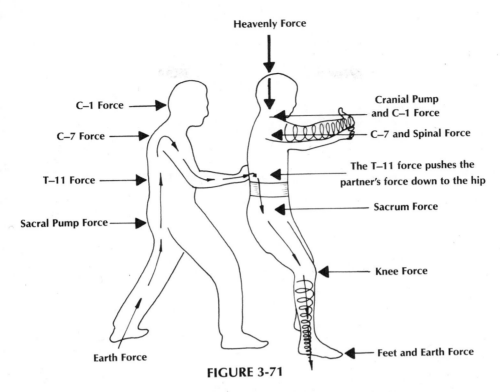

Heavenly Force

C–1 Force

C–7 Force

T–11 Force

Sacral Pump Force

Earth Force

Cranial Pump and C–1 Force

C–7 and Spinal Force

The T–11 force pushes the partner's force down to the hip

Sacrum Force

Knee Force

Feet and Earth Force

FIGURE 3-71

The partner's force is transferred down to the ground through the bone
structure by the force of T–11

aids in moving the energy to the upper body. Assume the position for Embracing the Tree, and pack with CHI as described. Your partner then pushes his fist against T–11 as you press back with that area of the spine. The work is done by the spine, not by the whole body. (Figure 3–71) Do not lean towards your partner.

7. Strengthening C–7

C–7, or the seventh cervical vertebra, is considered the point at which all the tendons of the body join together. By strengthening this part, the tendons, the fasciae and the neck will be strengthened. The C–7 also is the junction point of hand and spinal cord power.

Assume the position for Embracing the Tree and pack with CHI pressure as described. Your partner then pushes his palm (not his fist) against C–7 as you press back with C–7. Hold this position for as long

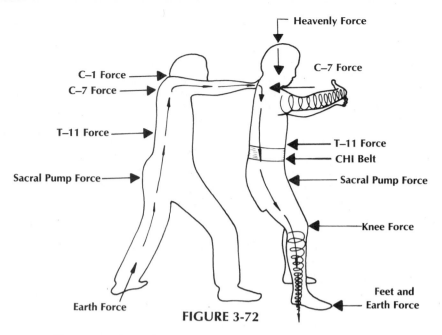

FIGURE 3-72

The partner's force is transferred down to the ground through the bone
structure by the force of C–7

as you can. (Figure 3–72) Your partner should coordinate with you
when you are ready to release.

8. Strengthening the Cranial Pump

The cranial pump has long been regarded by Taoists as a major
pump for the circulation of energy throughout the body. It has been
previously mentioned that minute movements at the joints of the
eight cranial bones occurs during breathing. Cranial movement stim-
ulates the production and function of the cerebrospinal fluid surrounding the brain and spinal cord. The cerebrospinal fluid is necessary for normal nerve and energy patterns in the entire body.
Strengthening the cranial pump can increase energy and alleviate
symptoms such as headaches, sinus problems, visual disturbances
and neck problems.

Assume the position for Embracing the Tree and pack with CHI
pressure. Clench the teeth, tighten the neck and contract the cranium
by squeezing the muscles around the skull and pressing the tongue
tightly to the roof of the mouth to activate the cranial bones. Push
back as your partner pushes his palm against C–1 at the base of the
skull. (Your partner should use his palm, not his fist.) (Figure 3–73)

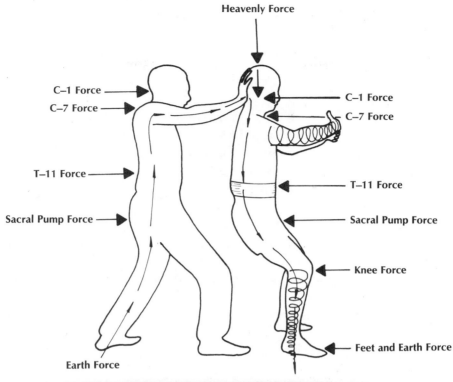

Heavenly Force

C–1 Force

C–7 Force

C–1 Force

C–7 Force

T–11 Force

T–11 Force

Sacral Pump Force

Sacral Pump Force

Knee Force

Feet and Earth Force

Earth Force

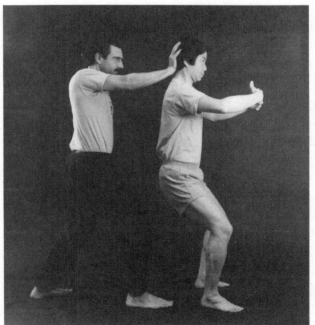

FIGURE 3-73

The partner's force is transferred down to the ground through the bone
structure by the force of C–1

9. Building Up Rootedness

a. Left and right side Rooting Practice

Assume the stance for Embracing the Tree and pack with CHI energy as described. Your partner stands to one side of you, placing one hand on your shoulder and the other on your hip. Your partner pushes you lightly, gradually increasing to full force. If you are well-rooted, the force of the push will flow right through your bone structure, down to the feet and into the earth. (Figure 3–74) If you have learned to direct and absorb energy through the bone structure and into the soles of the feet, you will be able to receive the powerful healing energy created by the blending of your energy, your partner's energy and raw earth energy. Your practice should have acquainted you with the flow of energy that goes down through the feet into the earth and then back out of the earth, up through the feet into you, while at the same time you are using the rest of the foot to "claw" against the floor.

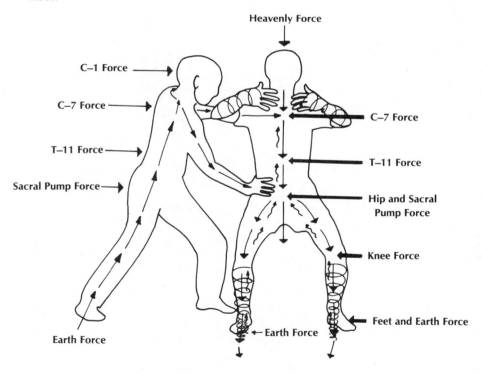

FIGURE 3–74

The partner's force is transferred down to the ground through the bone structure by the left and right side rooting practice

Have your partner push on the left side first, and then the right. Do the Energizer Breathing and resume the stance again. Have your partner push the right side. In the beginning, you will be tight and tense. You will need to use Packing Process Breathing, holding the breath to hold your structure together. As your practice improves and you are able to control and pack the energy, it will not be necessary to hold the breath since you will be able to maintain the structure and rooting in a relaxed manner without packing and without tensing the muscles at all. If the shoulder and spine are not joined together, you will fall. (Figure 3–75)

b. Front rooting

Front rooting is primarily training the front structure to root more solidly to the ground, especially the hands, the ribs, the front of the legs, and the soles and toes. Many people will find it hard to do any rooting to the ground at all. You must feel the force of your partner pass to the shoulder, to the scapula, to the spine, to the sacrum, to the hip and to the leg as one line.

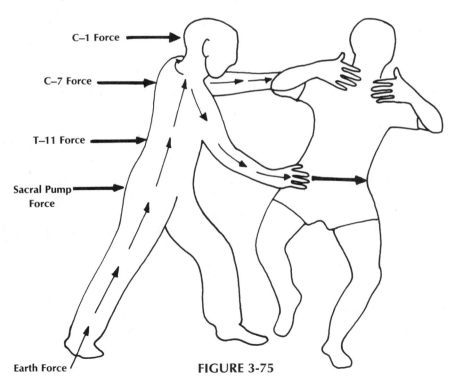

C–1 Force

C–7 Force

T–11 Force

Sacral Pump Force

Earth Force

FIGURE 3-75

If the force is not grounded, the force does not pass through the structure
and the body falls

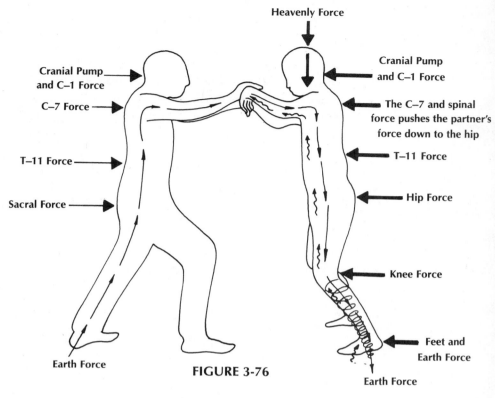

FIGURE 3-76

Front Pushing and Transferring the Force to the Ground

Assume the Embracing the Tree stance. Your partner pushes you on both wrists with both of his palms. (Figure 3–76) Front rooting is very hard and takes a lot of practice. In the beginning it is difficult, so apply only a small force and gradually increase. This will open the leg channels and hand channels and join them together. C–7 and the spinal cord play a very important role in the front rooting practice.

c. One legged stance rooting

Stand on one leg and circle out the opposite arm. Sink the chest. Feel how the arms and legs are in one line, connecting together. Sink so that the structure is joined. When your partner pushes, you can guide your partner's force down to the ground. (Figure 3–77)

d. Force transfer

The arm, the scapula, the spine, and the leg become one line, similar to a stick sticking into the ground. (Figure 3–78) If you try to push

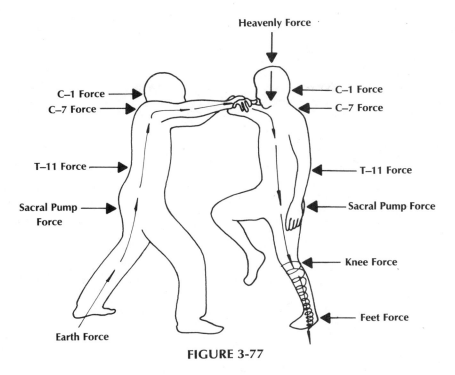

FIGURE 3-77

One Legged Stance and Transferring the Force to the Ground

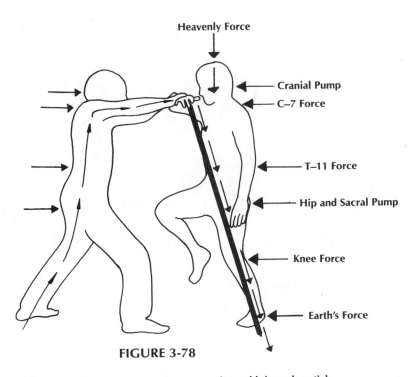

FIGURE 3-78

The force transfers through the bone structure as it would through a stick
sticking into the ground

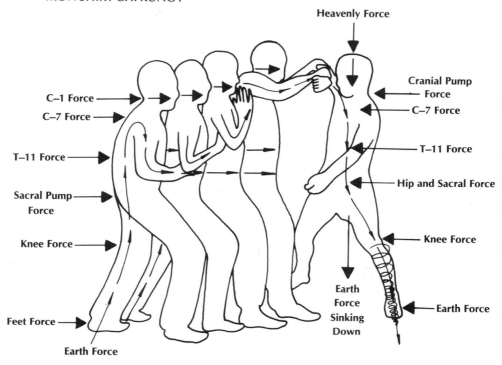

Heavenly Force

Cranial Pump Force

C–1 Force

C–7 Force

C–7 Force

T–11 Force

T–11 Force

Hip and Sacral Force

Sacral Pump Force

Knee Force

Knee Force

Feet Force

Earth Force Sinking Down

Earth Force

Earth Force

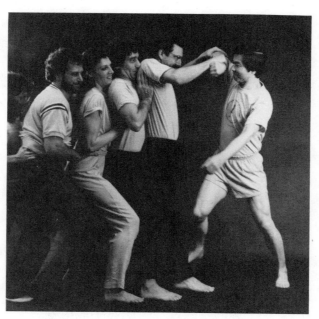

FIGURE 3–79

The partners' forces are transferred down to the ground through the bone structure because the body is properly aligned with the ground on the end that is sticking into the ground, all the force is transferred to the ground. If the fasciae and tendons are not as strong as possible, the whole structure will break when pushed.

e. Rooting against people—force transferred by bone structure to the ground

When your partner pushes you, do not lean towards him. Trust your structure and feel the whole body join into one piece. Feel the bones like sponges absorbing the force and passing it along the bone structure to the ground. When you feel the force, open the knee a little and feel the knees connected to the earth. Feel the energy pass to the ground.

When someone pushes you, he passes the force to you. The tendency as your partner pushes you is to counter the force by pushing the elbows out. This action moves you out of alignment. Therefore, when you feel the energy come at you from the side of your body, keep the elbow down and redirect the force back to the scapula and to the spine. The force, then, will not push you out of alignment.

When you are good at aligning all of the joints together, no matter where the force directed at you comes from, you will be able to re-direct it down to the earth, rather than let it break your alignment.

The principle of rooting is to become like a stick. The stick is most powerful when positioned at a 45 degree angle. When you push the end of the stick from a right angle, the force will go into the earth. If your body alignment is joined with the earth, when the force comes, it will go right through you and into the earth. The stick is not what is powerful; it is the earth behind it which has the power. Naturally, the stick has to be strong to pass the force. (Figure 3–79) The foot, the leg, the knee can all be adjusted to be like a 45 degree angle stick

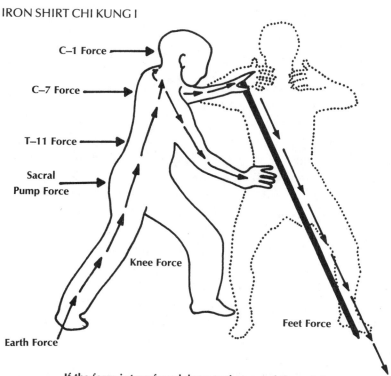

C–1 Force

C–7 Force

T–11 Force

Sacral
Pump Force

Knee Force

Feet Force

Earth Force

If the force is transferred down to the ground through the
bone structure, it is as if the partner is pushing a
stick into the ground

FIGURE 3-80

protruding from the earth. No matter what position you are in, you must always bear in mind that your body must be aligned with the ground, so that the force will not stay in the joints but can pass through the bone to the ground. (Figure 3–80)

B. Collecting CHI Energy After Practice

1. Preventing Side Effects

After each practice, stand silently erect for a few moments. Concentrate your attention on the navel, collecting the CHI there. As the CHI sinks down, stroke the chest from top to bottom with the palms

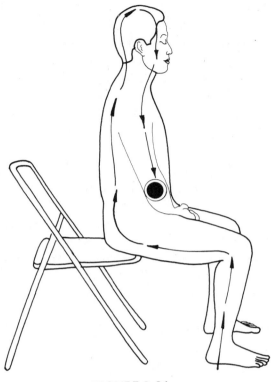

FIGURE 3-81

Collect the energy at the navel

of the hands. This prevents congestion of the chest and heart, as well as other side effects, such as heartburn, headache and eye pain. Move your hands to release the congestion and walk around until you feel the energy settle down.

After practicing Iron Shirt, take time to do the Microcosmic Orbit Meditation, also called the "Awaken Healing Energy" meditation, as described in Chapter 2. During your Iron Shirt Practice, you generate tremendous energy which tends to flow up and become trapped in the brain and the chest, especially in the heart. With practice, you will be able to direct the energy down to the navel from all sides and collect it there. (Figure 3–81) As your practice of Iron Shirt progresses, you will open up the navel area more for the storage of energy to be utilized in the higher spiritual practice.

2. Sitting and Standing Positions for Collecting Energy

When you have finished the Iron Shirt Practice, you should sit down to collect the energy that you have built up.

Sit on the edge of a chair using your sitting bones to find that delicate point of balance which will help hold you erect. (Figure 3-82(a). Men should sit far enough forward to allow the scrotum to hang freely. Women should also sit forward and should keep genitalia covered to avoid energy loss. The back must be comfortably erect, the head bowed slightly forward.

Stand straight, touch the tongue to the palate, and put the palm on the navel. (Figure 3-82(b)) Smile down to the organs and bring the energy to them. Let the energy circulate in a circle, starting from the navel down to the perineum and up the sacrum, to the spine, to the top of the crown and down the third eye to the tongue, to the heart, to the solar plexus, and to the navel. Do this several times and collect CHI in the navel by circulating it 36 times outward and 24 times inward to the navel.

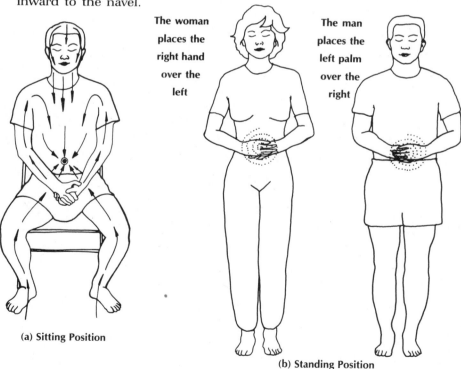

The woman places the right hand over the left

The man places the left palm over the right

(a) Sitting Position

(b) Standing Position

FIGURE 3-82

Sitting and Standing Position for Collecting Energy in the Navel

C. Illustrations of Postures

1. Holding the Golden Urn

Designed to strengthen the pinky and thumb fingers, Holding the Golden Urn joins the pinky fingers to a line which runs up and around the ears (at which location is housed one of the two major cranial bones), down the sides and to the small toes (Figure 3–83(a)), and strengthens the thumb line by joining it to the cranial bone, to the chest, to the navel and down to the big toes. (Figure 3–83(b)). These two lines are very important in holding the muscle tendons and bone structures together. When connected, these two tendons issue force on the sides and the front. Holding the Golden Urn is divided into two positions: the Yang Position and the Yin Position.

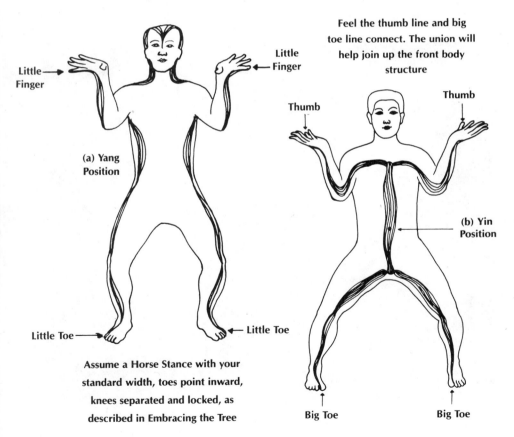

FIGURE 3-83

Holding the Golden Urn

a. Yang Position

Assume a Horse Stance with your standard width, toes point inward, knees separate and locked as mentioned above in Embracing the Tree. (Figure 3–84)

Bend your arms (as shown in the figure) so that your elbows, at a shoulders' width apart, drop and are forward vertically, causing your upper arms to be about 45 degrees away from your back and your forearms about 30 degrees out to your sides (not directly in front of your upper arms), with the wrists at 90 degree angles. For both hand positions of the Golden Urn, round the shoulders forward, then feel as if you are pressing up strongly, but without actually moving the arms. The chest sinks down slightly in response to the scapulae pulling around. In the Yang position, your hands are spread, palms down, with a pull exerted on the tendons of your fifth fingers (pinkies), so that the backs of your hands make a flat surface upon which you

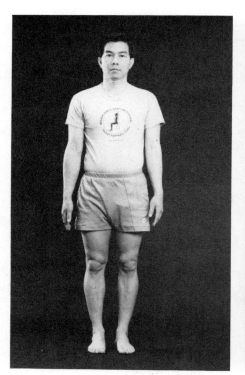
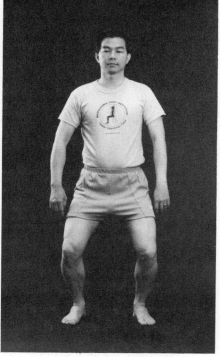

FIGURE 3-84

Holding the Golden Urn—Yang Position

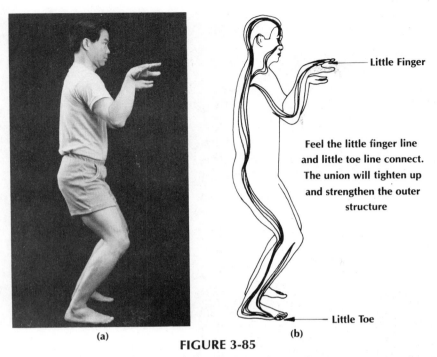

Little Finger

Feel the little finger line
and little toe line connect.
The union will tighten up
and strengthen the outer
structure

Little Toe

(a)   (b)

FIGURE 3-85

Holding the Golden Urn—Yang Position, Side View

could support a large "Golden Urn". (Figure 3–85(a)) (The spread fingers with the outward pull felt in the pinkies produce a bracing action that enables you to sustain considerable weight.) The tendon lines that are used here connect the small toes and small fingers, putting more force and energy in the small fingers and small toes. Small fingers are weak and seem useless but, when strenghtened, will give power to the whole structure. (Figure 3–85 (b)) The diagram shows the meridians of the fifth finger tendons joining the fifth toe tendons. This tightens and strengthens the entire outer structure.

b. Practice

In the Golden Urn we use one breath, but many inhalations. This means continue to inhale until you are out of breath, then exhale. This is regarded as one breath.

Your tongue should be at your palate throughout to keep the energy flowing safely.

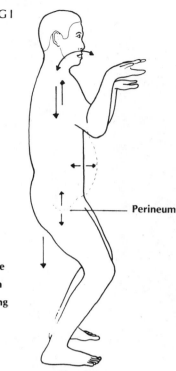

Perineum

Begin Holding the
Golden Urn with
Energizer Breathing

FIGURE 3-86

(1) Start with Energizer Breathing, nine to eighteen times. (Figure 3–86) Exhale and flatten the stomach. Inhale and pull up the left and right side of the anus. Bring the CHI to pack, circle and wrap around the kidneys.

(2) Inhale and pack the CHI in the lower abdominal area, contracting the anus, and pull up more on the urogenital diaphragm. Feel energy draw up from the soles of the feet to the sacrum.

(3) Inhale, packing to the sexual organs. Tilt the sacrum back to create a suction and pull the back part of the anus toward the sacrum.

(4) Inhale and pack the CHI at the sacrum. Tilt the sacrum back.

(5) Inhale and pack up to T–11, tilting or pushing the T–11 to the back (or use a wall as a guide and push the T–11 to the wall) until you feel like a flexed bow. The power of the bow is felt as the T–11, in being pushed back, creates a tension in joining together with the C–7. Inflate the back with CHI pressure, contract the anus and pull up the urogenital diaphragm. Feel the energy rise from the soles (K–1) to the T–

11. Feel a big band or CHI Belt stretching from the T–11 to the Door of Life and then towards the navel and lower abdomen.

(6) Inhale, contracting the anus more and lifting the genitals, drawing more energy up from the feet and packing it into the kidneys and C–7. (Figure 3-87) Tilt the C–7 to the back (use the wall as a guide and push the C–7 to the wall) until you feel the C–7's strong connection to the T–11 and sacrum. Feel the full strength of the flexed bow as the CHI inflates the entire neck. Hold for a while.

(7) Inhale and pull up more, tighten the neck and squeeze the cranial bones. Clench the teeth and press the tongue up to the roof of the mouth. Inhale. Pull the energy up to the base of the skull and squeeze more in the cranial bones. Tilt the neck to the back (use a wall as a guide by pushing the neck toward the wall). Feel the neck and the base of the skull have a strong connection with C–7, T–11, the sacrum, the knees, and the feet, and feel them become one flexed bow of strength. Inhale more and tighten, bringing energy up to the crown.

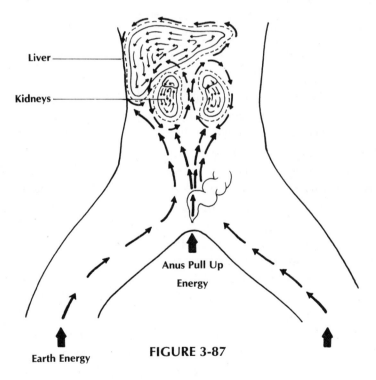

Liver

Kidneys

Anus Pull Up

Energy

Earth Energy

FIGURE 3-87

Draw the energy from the feet up to pack and wrap the kidneys

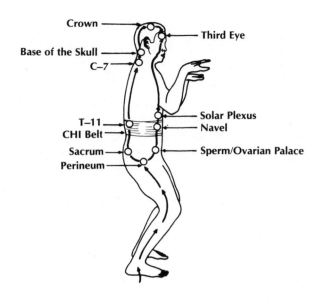

Crown — Third Eye
Base of the Skull
C-7
T-11 — Solar Plexus
CHI Belt — Navel
Sacrum
Perineum — Sperm/Ovarian Palace

FIGURE 3-88

The Flow of Energy During Holding the Golden Urn

(Figure 3–88) Stop for a while, and exhale. Relax. Follow with the Yin Position.

c. Yin Position

(1) Turn the hands over, palms up, and rotate the hands outward so that the thumbs now pull back and out to the ears with the wrists at 90 degree angles. Feel the stretch of the wrist tendons by locking the elbows and the wrists when turning the hands. The elbows sink in. The scapulae are rounded. When you stretch the thumbs, you are stretching the tendons. This is the Yin position. (Figure 3–89(a) and (b))

(2) Breathe normally. You should feel the energy rush up and over the head, into your arms and down the front of the body to the navel. Concentrate on the solar plexus. Make sure the energy is flowing down from the tongue to the solar plexus and navel along the Microcosmic Orbit. Considering an inhalation and an exhalation as one cycle, do nine cycles. Exhale more and inhale less. This is called Yin breathing. It will help to bring the energy down the front more easily.

(3) Yin Position—side view (Figure 3–90): When the thumb and toe

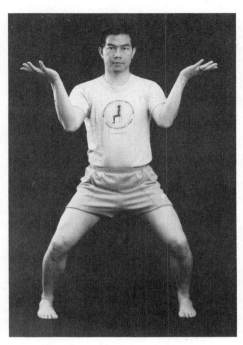

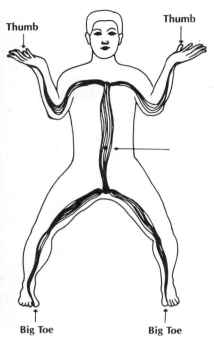

(a) Holding the Golden Urn—
Yin Position, Front View

FIGURE 3-89

(b) Thumbs and Big Toes Line

Thumb

Thumb

Big Toe

Big Toe

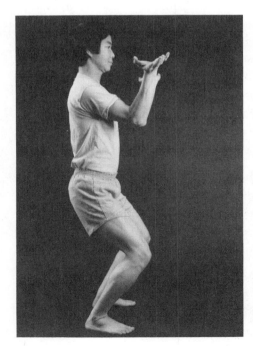

FIGURE 3–90

Holding the Golden Urn—
Yin Position, Side View

lines are linked together, they will connect all the muscles, tendons, bones, and the spinal cord to operate as a single structure. This will help the rooting power in the front energy line.

In the Yin position, the flow runs from the thumbs to the upper arms, and the big toes connect with the knees, navel and thumbs. The thumbs connect with the lungs and with tendons that run down the torso and the front of the legs to the big toes.

d. Holding the Golden Urn—Rooting Practice

Using his thumb and index finger, your partner will press against your wrist and place another hand on your hip. Start with the left side, then do the right side.

e. Rootedness

(1) Yang Position Rooting: Assume the Yang position and pack in energy to the abdomen, the spinal cord, and up to the neck. Feel the strength of the spine, as a flexed bow. Now, brace your tendon lines by extending your pinky fingers out very strongly. Have your partner attempt to push you out of the stance by gradually pressing against the wrist and the hip. (Figure 3–91(a))

(2) Yin Position Rooting: With your bodies connected in Yang Position Rooting, turn your hands over and you can transform the force to the ground through the bone structure. The thumbs link with the big toes. You must feel the thumb gaining force. The whole front line, starting from the thumb and continuing to the arm, hand, front of the head, ear, arm pit, front of the hip, and the leg to the big toe, is connected and pitted against your partner's force. Have your partner attempt to push you out of the stance by gradually pressing against the wrist and the hip.

f. Back and Front Pushing

Back pushing strengthens the whole spinal cord, the pinky fingers and small toes, and the back fasciae. Return to the Yang position. Be sure to press the big and small toes down, and feel that you are exerting force on the small toes and on the small fingers. Have your partner push from the back while you assume the stance. (Figure 3–91(b))

tain the stance and have your partner push your chest. (Figure 3–91(c))

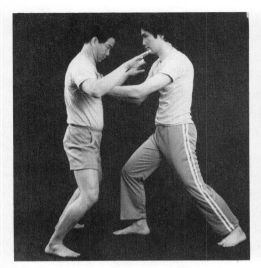

(c) Front pushing will increase the thumb and tendon power

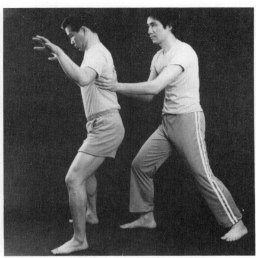

(b) Back Pushing

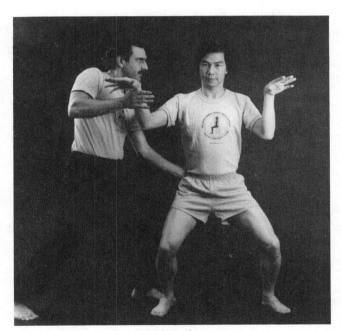

(a) Side Pushing

FIGURE 3-91

Front, Back and Side Pushing

When the tendons are used properly, less effort is needed to maintain good structure. In the Yang position, notice the feeling of support along the tendon lines.

Exhale and relax. Begin by assuming the Yang position. Quickly pack in energy to the whole back and to the neck. Move into the Yin position by turning the hands over and pulling the thumbs back. Feel the relationship between the thumbs and big toes. Keep this awareness as your partner pushes you in the Yin position.

2. SUMMARY of Holding the Golden Urn

a. Yang Position

(1) Stand with feet a knee-to-toe length apart; sink the elbows; hold the hands open at shoulder level with the palms down; lock the wrists; hold the hands at a 45 degree angle to the forearms; stretch out the pinky fingers so that you feel the energy in the small fingers; and feel the connection between the small fingers and the small toes. (The muscle-tendon meridian from the pinky fingers goes up the arms, up the side of the face and around the ears, down the outside of the arms, through the scapulae, down into the sacrum, and down the outside of the legs to the small toes.)

(2) Breathe below the navel (lower abdominal breathing).

(3) Exhale, pull up on the genitals, the perineum and the anus, locking the knees and feet.

(4) Inhale and pack in the navel.

(5) Inhale and pack the middle abdomen.

(6) Inhale and pack the lower abdomen.

(7) Inhale, tilt the sacrum, and pack the sacrum.

(8) Inhale and pack T–11 and the kidneys' areas.

(9) Inhale, lock the neck, bring the energy up to C–7, and inflate the neck.

(10) Inhale to the Jade Pillow, squeeze the skull and the temple bones.

(11) Inhale to the crown.

b. Yin Position

(1) Exhale, turning the hands with the wrists locked, energize the thumbs, and bring the energy down. (The route from the thumbs goes down the inside of the arms to the collar bones, to the sides of the

sternum, down to the navel and spreads out to both legs, down the inside of the thighs to the lower legs and to the big toes.)

(2) Place the hands over the navel, bring the feet together, and relax.

(3) Practice the Bone Breathing Process.

3. The Golden Turtle and the Water Buffalo

People with high blood pressure should consult a doctor before attempting this posture.

This posture energizes the toes and all the tendons of the toes and the fasciae of the thigh and the legs and strengthens the back fasciae, spinal cord, sacrum, kidneys, adrenal glands, neck and the head.

This position is called the "turtle back". The back will be energized like a blown-up balloon.

The workout given by this pose is equivalent to a headstand, but rather than blood flowing to the head, CHI is directed to the head, making it easier to direct and circulate the increased blood flow downwards.

Due to weakness in the thighs or tight hip joints, you may feel excessive strain when you first begin to practice the Turtle/Buffalo positions, even if you are not sinking very deeply into the position. If this is the case, practice with a chair or table in front of you on which to rest the arms. This support will enable you to gradually work into the position without straining yourself. (Figure 3–92)

Note that the back is straight and parallel to the floor

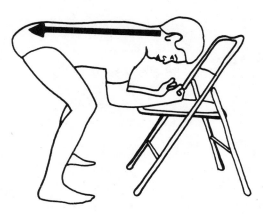

FIGURE 3-92

The Turtle/Buffalo Position—Side View

It is very important to keep the back straight and parallel to the floor. It may be difficult to feel when this is happening at first. Practice occasionally in front of a mirror to help develop the inner feeling of this occurrence.

a. The Golden Turtle Immersing in Water—Yang Position

(1) Place the legs in the standard stance.

(2) Begin Energizer Breathing. Breath in and out nine to eighteen times, inhaling more, exhaling less. When exhaling, keep the abdomen flattened to the spine.

(3) Inhale. Tighten the fists, fold the forearms against the upper arms, round the back, and sink the chest. Exhale and bend forward with the back straight so that the line made from the coccyx to the top of the head is horizontal to the floor. (Figure 3–93)

(4) Keep the forearms folded onto the upper arms, resting in front of the chest. (Figure 3–94) Keep the armpits open to make a space big enough to accommodate an object about the size of a pigeon egg. Round the scapulae. The back feels like a turtle and is energized with CHI.

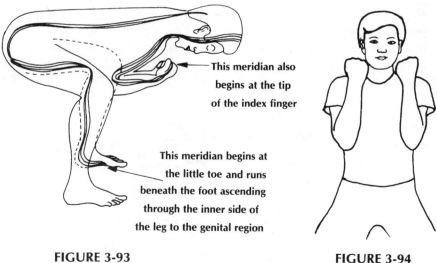

This meridian also
begins at the tip
of the index finger

This meridian begins at
the little toe and runs
beneath the foot ascending
through the inner side of
the leg to the genital region

FIGURE 3-93

FIGURE 3-94

The Muscle-Tendon Meridian
in the Turtle Position

Position of Forearms During
the Golden Turtle

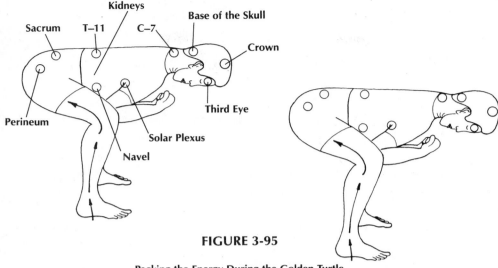

FIGURE 3-95

Packing the Energy During the Golden Turtle

(5) Lock the sacrum and open the knees so that you can feel the weight of the body sink down to the hips, to the knees, to the feet and, finally, to the ground. The spine should be horizontal to the ground. Pull the energy into the groin area where the sexual energy is. Tuck in the chin and set the neck firmly in position. Press the elbows against the inside of the knees. With the elbows, press out against the knees, while the knees press in, equalizing the force. Neither should press harder than the other.

(6) Inhale ten percent and pack the energy in the abdominal region (navel). Hold until you are out of breath.

(7) Inhale and pack down to the lower abdomen.

(8) Inhale, pack at the perineum and pull on the sexual organs more tightly. Pull the Mother Earth energy up to the perineum.

(9) Inhale, pack at the sacrum and tilt the sacrum. Pull up the sex organs more firmly.

(10) Inhale, pack at T–11, the kidneys and adrenal gland areas. Tilt the T-11. Feel the entire spine as a fully flexed bow. Inflate the lower back with CHI pressure and energize the kidneys.

(11) Inhale, pack at C–7. Tighten the neck and the cranial bones. Clench your teeth.

(12) Inhale up to the crown. (Figure 3–95)

See Figure 3–96 (a) through (k) for additional exercises utilizing the Golden Turtle Position.

189

FIGURE 3-96

The following are additional exercises in the Turtle position. For maximum results, they should be practiced in the sequence given, repeating the entire sequence three times

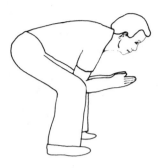

(a) From the basic stance, with the outside edges of the feet parallel, squat down, placing the elbows between the knees with the palms together. Keep the back as parallel to the floor as possible and your eyes looking up. Press out with the elbows resisted by the knees. Press and resist for two seconds, then release and relax

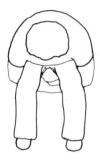

(b) Hook both elbows around the outside of the legs with the forearms behind the knees (Front View)

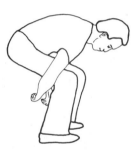

(c) Side View

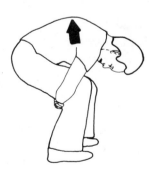

(d) Clasp the forearm or elbow with the opposite hand. Bring the head and tail down and toward each other as if looking at your tail. This is very important for protecting your back. Let the shoulder blades spread and the T-11 become your uppermost point

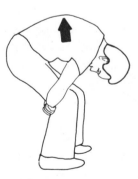

(e) Pull up strongly, forcing the T–11 and mid-back upwards against the resistance of the thighs, head and sacrum. Pull and resist for only two seconds. Relax

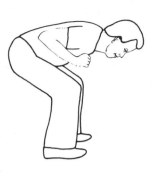

(f) Unlock the arms and bring them to the sides with the forearms rotated so that the palms face the floor. Pull the shoulder blades together

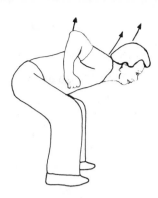

(g) Bring the elbows and head up

(h) Press the elbows up hard, lifting the head and looking forward while pressing the sternum forward. Hold two seconds. Relax (Side View)

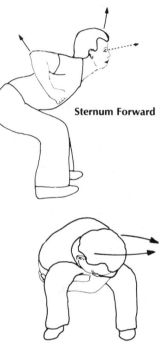

Sternum Forward

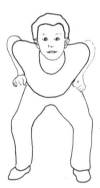

(i) Front View

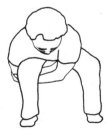

(j) Lock the arms around one knee, clasping the elbows behind the knee while looking at the floor

(k) Keep looking at the floor while you pull your ear and tail to the side opposite the knee you are holding, resisting with that knee. After two seconds, place the hands on the floor, wag the tail to relax, and then repeat the exercise on the opposite side. Again, wag the tail to relax the spine. During the exercise, the whole column from tail to head should form a curve like the letter "C" parallel to the floor and you should feel a stretching on the sides of the spine and the neck

b. The Water Buffalo—Yin Position

(1) When you have packed the energy to the head, exhale and look slightly up by moving the neck up, thereby relieving the tension of the lock in the neck. Extend the arms down in front of you with the backs of the hands facing frontwards and the fingertips touching the perineum and the anus or touching the ground. Keep the groin (genital area) open. (Figure 3–97)

(2) Practice the open groin breathing process. (Figure 3–98) Relax, keeping the tongue up. Inhale less, exhale more, breathing right into the groin area. In this position, the groin is open and you can breathe down to the lower part of the body which greatly energizes the sexual organs and increases circulation tremendously. Breathe easily and feel the energy descend to the navel and perineum, activating and strengthening the circulation of the lower abdomen. The urogential and pelvic diaphragms, which hold the sexual organs, bladder, and large and small intestines in place, become activated as well.

When your breath has normalized, close your eyes. Slowly bring yourself to a standing position. Remember, when you get up, do so very slowly to avoid dizziness. Stand erect. Work up some saliva and, tightening the neck, swallow down to the navel with a guttural sound. Feel the saliva shoot down to the navel and burn with CHI power. Normalize breathing and place the hands over the navel. Collect CHI in the navel.

Practice Bone Breathing to absorb CHI into the bones. Meditate standing for a while. If you wish, work on circulating the CHI in the Microcosmic Orbit. Then walk around, shaking out the legs and brushing down the chest.

c. Turtle Position—Rooting Practice

In the Turtle Position, the elbows are held in tightly, pressed against both thighs so that you can feel the energy concentrated in the groin area. The spine is horizontal to the ground. (Figure 3–99) Pack CHI along the whole back. Have your partner stand on the left side with his one hand on your shoulder and his other hand on your hip. (Figure 3–100) When your partner pushes you, lock the sacrum. Open the knees slightly and adjust the feet to align the force of your partner down to the ground. Become one with the earth. Gradually push and increase to whatever pressure you can take. The bone

Note that the back is straight

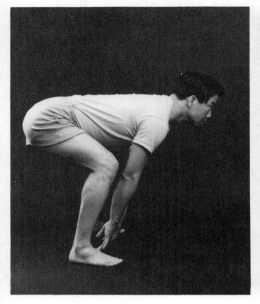

FIGURE 3-97

Buffalo—Right Side View

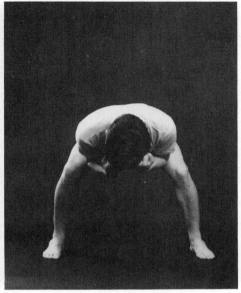

FIGURE 3-99

Turtle—Front View

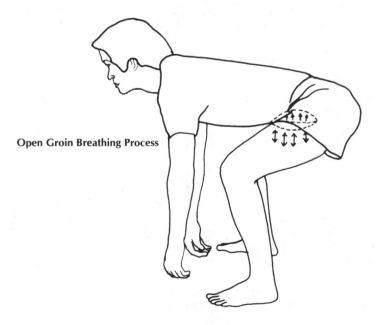

Open Groin Breathing Process

FIGURE 3-98

Buffalo—Left Side View

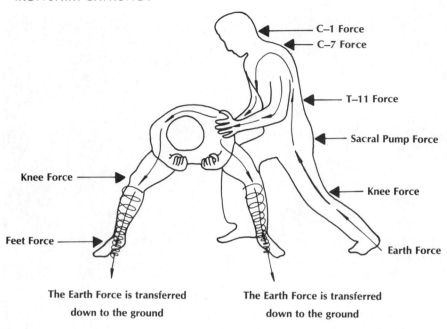

C–1 Force

C–7 Force

T–11 Force

Sacral Pump Force

Knee Force

Knee Force

Feet Force

Earth Force

The Earth Force is transferred
down to the ground

The Earth Force is transferred
down to the ground

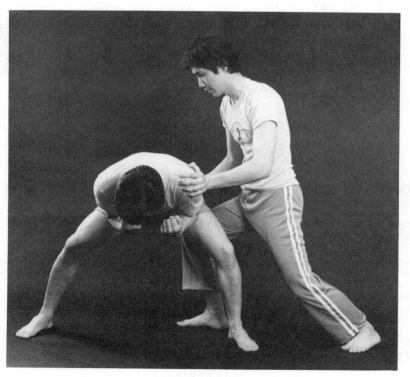

FIGURE 3-100

Rooting Practice During the Golden Turtle—Left Side Position

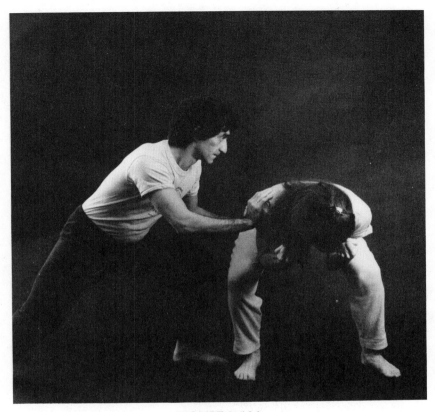

FIGURE 3-101

The Golden Turtle—Right Side Position

structure is like a sponge absorbing the force and transferring it to the ground.

Your partner should not continue to push when you are out of breath and about to rest. Once you become adept in this practice and you feel your body's structure as one piece, you will feel the muscles relax and find no need for Packing Breathing. If you simply concentrate on the CHI flow and relax, the force will pass through the bone structure.

Change sides and let your partner push you gradually. (Figure 3–101) The purpose is not to push you over, but to let you feel where the force comes from so that you can redirect the force to the earth.

When the force is started gradually, you are able to feel where the force is going, permitting you to re-align or relax that part to let the force pass through.

Always balance out both sides by having your partner push on both the left and right sides. Remember, one side is generally stronger than the other.

Once you can successfully redirect the force from any part of your body, you will start to know how to reabsorb the force from the earth. The force that your partner pushes you with, when directed to the earth, can be reabsorbed back from the earth and becomes more powerful than before. This energy can be used for self-healing, or to counteract your partner's pushes. In the higher level, you can pass that force to your partner to heal him or her as well.

After each pushing, go back to the Buffalo Position. The chin is up, the shoulders relax, the hands drop down to near the groin area, or touch the sexual organs to strengthen the pelvic and urogenital diaphram energy. Breathe deeply to the groin area to strengthen the sexual/creative energy.

The Turtle Position strengthens the whole back and spine. When your partner pushes from the left, you feel the force go from the left shoulder, pass the scapula to the spine, to the right scapula, down the spine to the hip, to the right thigh, the right leg and foot and down to the ground. At the same time, feel the sole breathing and "claw" down with the toes into the ground.

If the pressure is too much, the left foot will uproot. Push down the left foot by exerting more pressure on the hip down to the thigh and the leg.

Partners should be roughly equal in size, stature and strength for pushing.

d. Turtle/Buffalo—Front Rooting Practice

Your partner should place one hand on each shoulder and gradually push you in order to strengthen the frontal aspect of this posture. (Figure 3–102) To maintain this difficult position, you must gradually feel the connection of the shoulders to the scapulae and the spine to the sacrum and the hips. Front rooting requires more practice. The soles and feet are very important to front rooting. With practice, you can maintain the feet's firm contact with the ground.

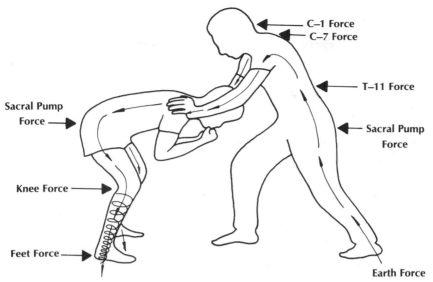

C–1 Force
C–7 Force

T–11 Force

Sacral Pump
Force

Sacral Pump
Force

Knee Force

Feet Force

Earth Force

The Force is transferred through the
bone structure into the ground

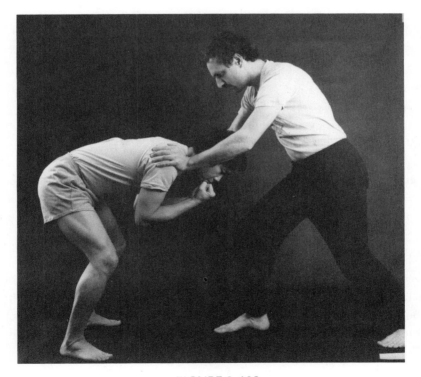

FIGURE 3-102

The Turtle/Buffalo—Front Rooting Practice

4. SUMMARIES of the Golden Turtle and the Water Buffalo

a. The Golden Turtle Immersing in Water (Yang Position)

(1) Place the tongue on the roof of the mouth.

(2) Practice lower abdominal breathing in a standing position.

(3) Bend forward with the back straight, bend the arms in close to the body, maintain the continuing line of the spine through the neck, and clench the fists.

(4) Inhale and pack to the navel.

(5) Inhale and pack to the middle abdomen.

(6) Inhale and pack to the lower abdomen.

(7) Inhale and pack to the perineum.

(8) Inhale and pack to the sacrum.

(9) Inhale and pack to the T–11.

(10) Inhale and pack to the C–7.

(11) Inhale and pack to the Jade Pillow.

(12) Inhale and pack to the crown of the head.

(13) Inhale and pack more along the back.

b. Water Buffalo Emerging from The Water (Yin Position)

(1) Exhale and regulate your breathing.

(2) Head and eyes should be looking up, but not straining. Keep the back level and extend the arms with the hands towards the ground slightly behind you or touching the groin area. Maintain the same back position.

(3) Practice lower abdominal breathing while focusing on the genital area.

(4) Close the eyes and gradually stand up. Put the hands on the navel area and collect the energy.

(5) Practice the Bone Breathing Process.

(6) Muscle Power Exercise.

5. The Golden Phoenix Washes Its Feathers

The Phoenix Position strengthens both sides of the ribs, from the armpits down to the sides of the hips and packs CHI pressure into all the major organs. On the left side, pack, wrap and squeeze the CHI to the left kidney, spleen, left lung, and heart; on the right side, you are

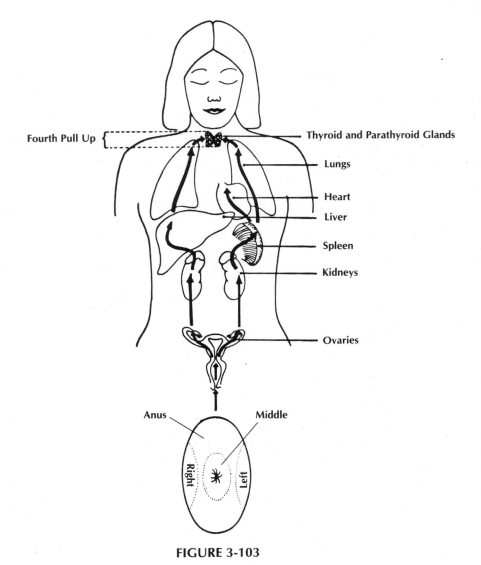

FIGURE 3-103

Wrap and squeeze CHI into all of the major organs

strengthening the right kidney, liver and right lung. (Figure 3–103)

The Phoenix Exercise also exercises the fingers, toes, tendons and the tongue (which is one of the main tendons of the body.) You will also exercise the tendons of the whole body. The pinky fingers are small, but can activate many tendons, especially along the sides of the body.

a. Practice

(1) Assume the Iron Shirt Horse Stance. (Figure 3–104(a)) Place your arms at your sides. Practice the Energizer Breathing to fan up the energy.

(2) Sweep the arms out to both sides and turn them over so that the wrists are straight. (Figure 3–104(b)) The palms begin to face up and are turned in towards the body, as though you were gathering something up under the armpits. The pinky fingers are pointed up toward the ceiling. (Figure 3–104(c)) Feel the pull of the tendons all the way up the arms to the ears, circling the ears, and down the sides of the body to the small toes. The scapulae are rounded. The neck muscles and the trapezius muscles are relaxed so that the hands and the arms are connected. The elbows are bent out to the side.

(3) Inhale while you pull up the left and right sides of the anus and bring the sexual energy from the testicles/ovaries to the kidneys. Pack in energy to the kidneys and to the level of the adrenals which are located at the top of the kidneys on about the same level as the solar plexus. Bring the palms up along the sides of the body, feeling the tension and the pull of the tendons on the insides of the arms up to the elbows, the pinkies and the thumbs.

(4) Inhale higher toward the armpits, pulling the sexual energy from the testicles/ovaries to the kidneys and up to the spleen on the left side and the liver on the right side. Hold and pack the CHI in the organs and then wrap the CHI around them. The palms still face up and the pinky fingers' tendons stretch toward the ceiling. Inhale and get closer to the armpits, pulling the sexual energy up to the heart, and to the lungs. Fill the lungs with CHI.

(5) Feel the whole rib cage and the armpits bulge up, filled with CHI. (Figure 3–104(d))

(6) When you get as close to the armpits as you can (Figure 3–104(e) and (f)), exhale while maintaining the contraction in the anus and the pull on the genitals. Rotate the hands medially. Face palms out (Figure 3–104(g)), pulling from the scapulae which are connected to the earth. The forearms are straight; the elbows are back; the wrists are locked; the knees are open. Push from the sternum to C–7 in order to feel the force come from the earth up into the heels, the sacrum, the spinal cord, the scapulae and the hands. (Figure 3–104(h)) As you

FIGURE 3-104   The Golden Phoenix Washes Its Feathers

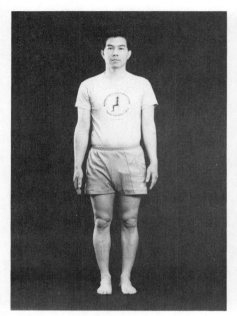

(a) Assume the Iron Shirt Horse Stance.
Place your arms at your sides.
Practice the energizer breathing
to fan up the energy

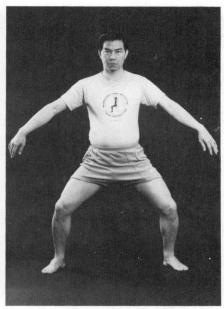

(b) Sweep the arms out to both sides
and turn them over so that the
wrists are straight

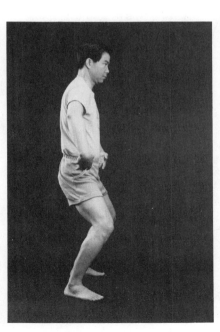

(c) The palms face up and are turned
in towards the
body with the pinky fingers pointed up

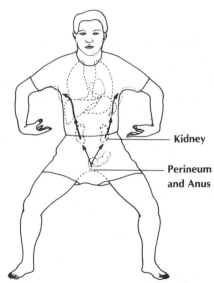

Kidney

Perineum
and Anus

(d) Pack the energy into the testicles/ovaries,
into the kidneys, then into
the spleen on the left side and the liver
on the right side. As you continue
to pack and pull the energy up to the
heart and to the lungs, you will feel
the rib cage bulge up

FIGURE 3-104

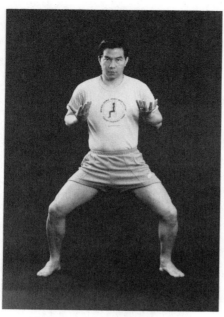

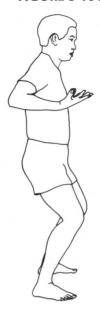

(e) The palms continue to face up

(f) Side View

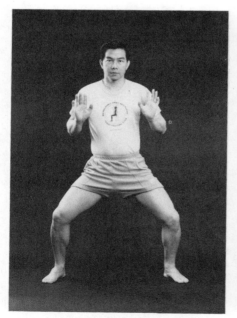

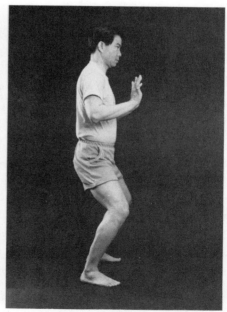

(g) Rotate the hands medially

(h) Push from the C–7 by sinking down the sternum and pressing towards the back

push, extend your arms and exhale using the First Healing Sound, the Lung Sound "SSSSSSSS". (A complete explanation of the Six Healing Sounds is provided in the book *Taoist Ways to Transform Stress into Vitality.*) From the palms of the hands to the heels of the feet you will feel like one piece. This is what is meant by "structure".

(7) When the arms are fully extended (Figure 3–104(i) and (j)), inhale and contract the middle of the anus and pull up the sexual organs. Feel the pull at the tip of the fingers of both hands. Gather the fingers to the thumbs and press them together in a small point by exerting more force on the pinky fingers (which should be in the middle with all the fingers pressed against it), and more force on the tips of all the fingers. (These finger positions are called "beaks"). (Figure 3–104(k)) Feel the pulling force in the anus and in the tips of the fingers combine into a single force.

(8) Inhale, pull the "beaks" inward from the elbows and contract the middle part of the anus. (Figure 3–104(l)) Feel the force of the anus and the sexual organ pull the "beaks" in.

(9) Inhale again, pulling the "beaks" closer to the body, further tightening the anus and genital area. (Figure 3–104(m)) While inhaling, pull the elbows and the wrists near the chest with the "beaks" pointed out.

(10) Exhale as you open the "beaks", extend the arms in front of you and then spread the fingers wide apart. (Figure 3–104(n)) Exhale, using the Second Healing Sound, the Kidney Sound "WOOOOOOO", and lower your arms in front of you, the heels of the hands leading the way with the action originating from the shoulders. (Figure 3–104(o)) When the arms have reached the sides of the hips, lock the elbows, keep the fingers spread apart and rotate the hands laterally out to each side. Flex the finger tendons out, especially the pinky fingers and the thumbs. Spread the toes out, especially the small toes. At the same time, extend the tongue out as far as you can to the chin. (Figure 3–104(p)) Direct your eyes to look at your nose. Feel the tongue and the sexual organs pull up as one line out to the tongue. Finally, turn the big toes and the heels inward, and then make the feet move towards one another by taking "steps" leading with the big toes and alternating with the heels until the feet come in together. This will exercise the feet tendons.

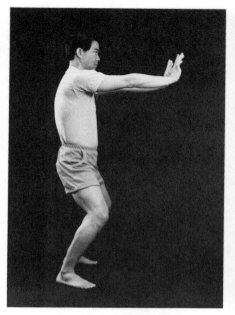

(i) Push and fully extend the arms. Side View

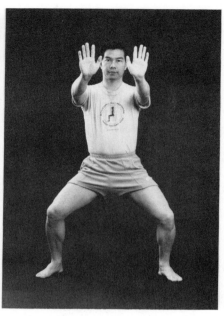

(j) Front view of arms fully extended.

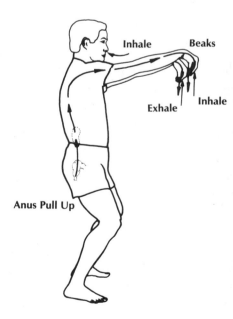

Inhale   Beaks

Exhale   Inhale

Anus Pull Up

(k) Gather the fingers and form "beaks"

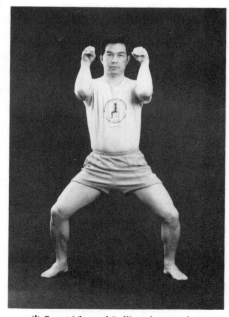

(l) Front View of Pulling the "Beaks"

FIGURE 3-104

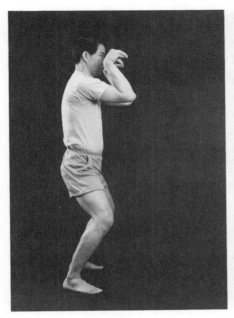

(m) Side View of Pulling the "Beaks"

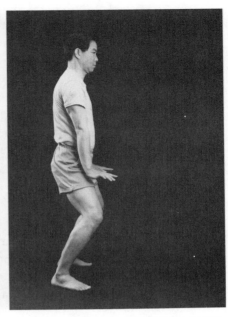

(n) Exhale. Release the "beaks". Press your arms against the front of your body

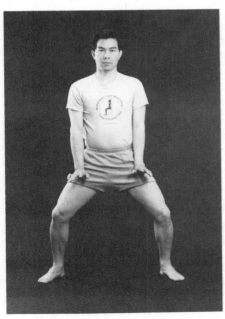

(o) Front View of the Arms Pressed Down

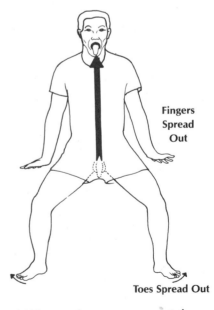

Fingers
Spread
Out

Toes Spread Out

(p) The sexual organs are connected to the tongue

Repeat steps (6) through (10). This time, however, replace the Lung Sound in Step (6) as you push your palms out straight in front of you with the Third Healing Sound, the Liver Sound "SHHHHHHH". Replace the Kidney Sound in Step (10) as you are lowering your arms in front of you, with the Fourth Healing Sound, the Heart Sound "HAWWWWWW". Repeat steps six through ten one more time. Replace the Lung and Liver Sounds in Step (6) with the Fifth Healing Sound, the Spleen Sound "WHOOOOOO". Replace the Kidney and Heart Sounds in Step (10) with the Sixth Healing Sound, the Triple Warmer Sound "HEEEEEE".

You should feel connected through the legs, spinal tendons, scapulae and arms.

(11) Spread the fingers apart and extend the arms. (Spreading the fingers enlists the use of tendon power.) Feel the force come out from the scapulae. Relax. Feel the CHI spread out to all the tendons of the hands, legs, and tongue. The tongue connects to the tendons.

b. Rooting Practice of the Golden Phoenix:
Feel the Force Transfer from the Hand to the Ground

Practice the Phoenix Exercise and extend the arms out. Lock the elbows. Lock the wrists. Round the scapulae. Pull up the middle anus and the genital area. Open the knees. Feel that the palms and feet are connected to the ground. Have your partner use his palms to hit your palms. If you are well connected and are relaxing the muscles of the neck, you will feel the force travel to the ground.

c. The Lift Up Connected Practice

This exercise requires a locked wrist and hand with the shoulders and scapulae connected while your partner tries to lift you up. Be cautious because you can be hurt in this practice.

Lower the arms, shoulders and scapulae while bringing the hands to the sides of the thighs. Place the palms down, draw the elbows back, lock the wrists, round the scapulae, and feel the connection with the spinal cord. Have your partner put one leg between your legs, his palms turned in against your palms and lift you up. (Figure 3–105) Find a partner who is your height. Make sure that you lock the elbows, the wrists and the scapulae, otherwise you can hurt your wrists or scapulae, and your partner will be unable to lift you.

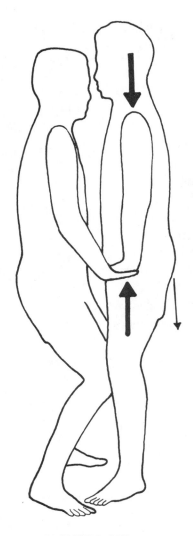

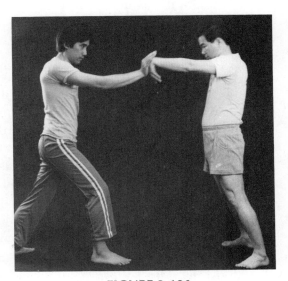

FIGURE 3-106

The "Beaks" Rooting Practice

FIGURE 3-105

The Lift Up Practice

d. "Beaks" Rooting Practice

Extend the arms and form "beaks", connecting the arms with the scapulae, the spine, the legs and the feet. Have your partner push the wrists, and feel the force trasnfer to the ground. (Figure 3–106)

6. SUMMARY of the Golden Phoenix Washes Its Feathers

a. Practice lower abdominal breathing in a standing position.

b. Place your arms in front of your body with the backs of the hands facing each other. Inhale and allow the arms to sweep out to your sides, pointing the fingers towards the ribs, and pull up the perineum and anus. Pack into the fasciae on the sides of the ribs and pack into the kidneys. Inhale, raising the hands up along the sides. Pack and wrap the CHI into the liver and spleen. Inhale once more raising the hands higher and pack and wrap the CHI into the lungs and heart.

c. Exhale, keeping the perineum and anus closed while pushing the hands out at shoulder level. Keep the wrists flexed.

d. Inhale and tighten at the perineum and anus. Form "beaks" with your fingers and bring them in toward the shoulders. Repeat twice more, raising the "beaks" a little higher each time.

e. Exhale, releasing the perineum and anus and lowering the arms while simultaneously straightening and locking the elbows and knees. When the hands are down with the wrists flexed, turn the hands out to the sides of the thighs and spread the fingers and toes out as much as possible. Thrust the tongue and pull up the anus and sexual organs.

f. Collect the CHI energy at the navel.

g. Practice the Bone Breathing Process.

7. Iron Bridge

The Iron Bridge is designed to strengthen the front and back fasciae. By stretching the fasciae from the pelvis to the neck and both sides of the rib cage in this exercise, you will greatly increase the flow of CHI between the fasciae and will tone up the front and back muscles considerably.

Arching the spine backwards greatly strengthens the lower spine, especially the lumbar region. By stretching the upper back and spine opposite to the normal direction of its curve, the backbend will help to lessen the often excessive forward curvature of the upper back, limber the shoulder joints, and open the chest. The point to remember is that the bend is from the upper back and not from the hip.

a. Iron Bridge Standing Position—Yang Position

This position will create a tremendous amount of CHI energy which will rise up the spine to the head.

(1) Stand, keeping the knees straight and the feet one foot apart. It is best for beginners if the feet are placed so that they point straight ahead along the second toes. If the toes turn out, there may be unnecessary compression in the lower spine, even if the knees are locked and the thighs and buttocks tightened. The thumbs and index fingers are touching each other and the remaining three fingers are held together. Keep the hands straight, low and slightly in front of the body.

(2) Begin abdominal breathing; exhale and flatten the abdomen. Inhale to full capacity. Bring the hands up and to the back, bend the elbows back, and place the palms up. (Figures 3-107(a) and (b)) Fingers should be about two inches apart and will rise close to the scapulae. This will open the sternum, activate the thymus, stretch the thyroid, the parathyroid, the chest and the side fasciae.

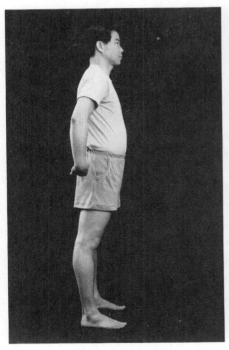 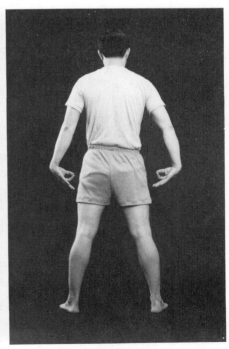

(a) Standing Position   (b) Back View of the Standing Position

FIGURE 3-107

The Iron Bridge

(3) Any accumulated tension in the chest and abdomen can be released. Hips stay over the feet. It is most important to arch the upper and middle back and not the hip. This will stretch the front fasciae. Excessive arching of the hip and lower spine can damage the discs between the vertebrae and pinch the nerves because of the excessive weight. Also, if the arching in the Iron Bridge is mostly from the lower spine, there will be much less stretching of the fasciae in the front of the torso. To keep the lower spine protected, it is necessary to arch the back strongly from the upper spine while firmly tightening the thighs and buttocks. By strongly tightening the thighs and buttocks, you can feel that you are squeezing the sacrum down, thus lessening the compression in the lower spine. The knees should be firmly locked and straight. This will allow the thighs and buttocks to be very firmly tightened.

(4) Clench the teeth. As you arch back, begin with the head. Rotate the head back from the upper neck, until you feel the front fasciae of the neck stretching. Do not let the head drop back as this is very bad for the neck vertebrae. If done properly, you will still feel that the neck is elongating upwards, even while it is rotated back. If there is any discomfort whatsoever, you are either practicing incorrectly or trying to stretch back too far.

Look back, locking and pulling the neck fasciae. (Figure 3–107(c)) As soon as the front of the neck has stretched properly, you will feel an automatic lifting at the chest which, as it stretches up, will then automatically stretch the abdomen. As the abdomen stretches, push the pelvis forward, keeping the thighs and buttocks very tight. As you stretch the chest, feel that the breastbone is being pulled forward and up. In this way, the upper back will be arching, rather than only the lower spine. (Figure 107(d))

If done properly, you will feel the fasciae being stretched from the groin up to the chest and the neck, pulling tight as a drum without having to arch very far back. (Figure 3–107(e)) If you are arching very far back, then you are inevitably overarching the lower spine. (Figure 3–107(f))

If your upper spine is not very flexible, or has a large forward curvature, then you may look as if you are hardly arched back at all when you first practice, though you will still be able to feel a stretch across

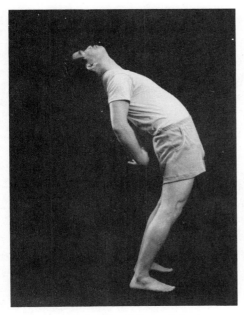

(c) Look back and pull the neck fasciae

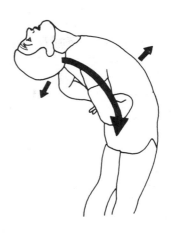

(d) Arch the upper and middle back

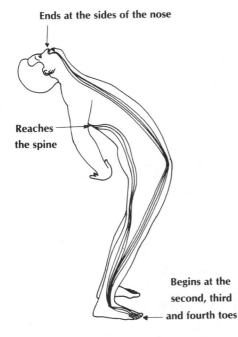

Ends at the sides of the nose

Reaches the spine

Begins at the second, third and fourth toes

(e) The stretch is felt beginning at the second, third and fourth toes up the back to the spine, and up the front until it ends at the sides of the nose

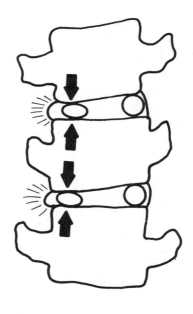

(f) Excessive arching of the hip and lower spine can damage the discs

FIGURE 3-107

the front torso. Remember that no matter how flexible you are, you will not arch very far back if you are practicing properly. It is a good idea to practice this upper body stretch while sitting until you can do it well before practicing in a standing position.

Remember also that if you bend too much initially, you may fall back. In the beginning, have a partner look after you when you bend back to steady you, if necessary.

(5) Squeeze the thumb and index fingers together and tighten the muscles of the arms and shoulders. This will stabilize your position.

(6) Hold your breath and maintain this position for 30 to 60 seconds.

b. Iron Bridge Resting Position—Yin Position

(1) Exhale. Straighten up and bring the arms to the front, maintaining the hand position, and slowly bend forward from the hip joint. The head is down and the hands are above or touching the ground. (Figure 3–108(a)) Do not force yourself.

(2) Adjust the tendons. In the beginning, do not bend too low and,

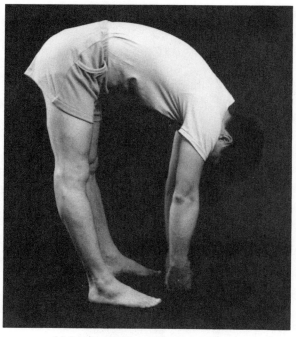

(a) Resting Position of the Iron Bridge

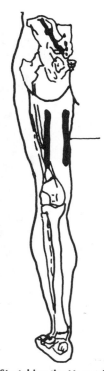

(b) Stretching the Hamstring

FIGURE 3-108

for additional comfort, you can slightly bend the knees. This is particularly important if you are practicing rooting in this position. If the knees are locked back, there will be strain in the knees. If you want to stretch farther forward, do not increase the forward curvature of the upper spine to do it. Stretch forward by letting the hamstring muscles at the backs of the thighs lengthen. (Figure 3–108(b)) If you are stretching forward vigorously, or are not very limber, bend the knees much more while stretching so that you can lay the whole abdomen firmly on the thighs. Then, test your flexibility by slightly straightening the knees, while keeping the abdomen on the thighs. Practicing in this way will guarantee that you are only stretching the lower spine and hamstrings, and not arching the upper spine.

Feel the CHI flow down to the head and back and down the tongue. The three fingers of each hand are nearly touching each other and you can feel the CHI flow from the right hand's middle finger to the left hand's middle finger, up the left arm to the spine, to the head and down to the navel. Stay relaxed until you feel the energy flow without obstruction. Some people may feel a certain vibration which gradually spreads throughout the body. Allow the vibration to occur for a while. Slowly stand up to avoid dizziness.

Maintain this position only for as long as you feel comfortable. It is quite strenuous and should be approached with moderation.

8. SUMMARY of the Iron Bridge

a. Standing Iron Bridge—Yang Position

(1) Assume the Horse Stance.

(2) Place hands at the sides of the body. Touch both thumbs and index fingers together, forming a circle. The other three fingers of each hand remain straight and touch one other.

(3) Breathe abdominally, inhale and look up at the ceiling. Arch back from the lower back, keeping the legs straight and the hips aligned over the legs to maintain balance.

b. Standing Iron Bridge—Yin Position

(4) When you feel you have had enough, exhale and bring the body slowly to a standing position.

(5) Bend the knees slightly in the beginning. Lower the head, and bend forward from the shoulders and chest, rounding the back.

(6) Relax the arms and allow them to dangle in front of you, maintaining the finger position with the fingers facing each other. Feel the CHI flow through each finger. If you can touch the ground, you can feel a certain connection of the CHI energy. Breathe normally.

(7) Come up very slowly from this position. You may feel dizzy at first. Stand still for a while, collect the energy, practice Bone Breathing and the muscle Power Exercise. Walk around, or lie down on your back and massage your belly from right to left to get your CHI circulating.

Additional Exercises: To strengthen the upper abdominals, do sit-ups with bent knees. The lower abdominals are strengthened by doing sit ups with your legs extended straight out in front of you, although it is recommended that this, as all exercises, not be excessively practiced.

c. Standing Iron Bridge—Rooting Practice

Assume the posture. Have your partner push very gently. Remember that the main arch is in the upper back. Be very careful in this Iron Bridge Rooting Practice. Your partner has to be aware that it is dangerous when you arch backwards. The back and spinal cord are vulnerable to injury in this position. Be careful to apply pressure gently to avoid hurting the spinal cord or falling down.

(1) Yin position Rooting Practice

While you are in the backbend position, your partner should put one hand on your back and one hand on your chest. (Figure 3–109(a)) As your partner slowly presses down, observe that you can take the force only for a few seconds. Bend forward to rest for a while and then practice rooting in the forward position.

(2) Yang position Rooting Practice

While you are bent forward, your partner should press his/her hands on your shoulders. (Figure 3–109(b)) You push up from the lower spine. He/she can use his/her entire body to press down. In this position you are exerting more force on the lower back. This will strengthen the lower spine, especially the lumbar region.

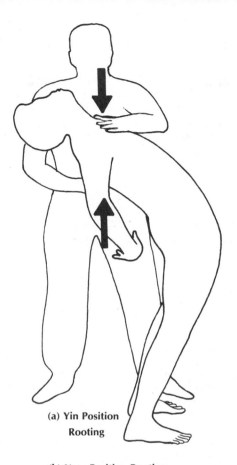

(a) Yin Position
    Rooting

(b) Yang Position Rooting

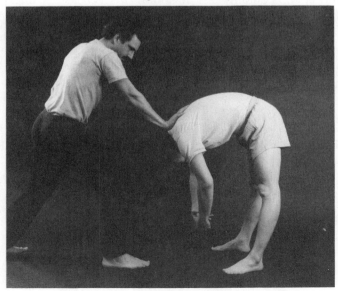

FIGURE 3-109

Iron Bridge Rooting

9. Iron Bar

The Iron Bar practice greatly strengthens the front and back fasciae and thus makes the spinal cord very strong. The spinal column consists of 24 vertebrae held together by tendons, fasciae and muscles. Normally, we do very little to exercise the vital spinal column. The Iron Bar exercise automatically adjusts all of the spinal column, strengthening it segment by segment.

a. Iron Bar Practice

(1) Place two chairs facing each other. Have your partner hold the chair at your head to keep it steady. If you do not have a partner, put one of the chairs against the wall.

(2) Put both hands palms down behind you on the floor and push yourself up on the chair. Put the feet and ankles on one chair, the head and shoulders on the other. Fold the hands across the belly. Straighten out the body, especially the lower back. With the toes pointed down and outward, you can feel a pull on the fasciae and tendons. (Figure 3–110(a) Make sure the lumbar region is straight, not bent. This will help to strengthen the front and back fasciae.

(3) If you initially feel that the Iron Bar is too difficult to do properly and comfortably, bring your arms back over your head onto the chair that your head is on. This makes it much easier to maintain a straight spine and is considerably less strenuous. As you feel stronger, gradually increase the amount of force with which you are pushing down the arms into the chair. When you can practice without pushing the arms down at all behind you, you are ready to move gradually to the final position with the hands resting over the navel.

(4) Place both hands on the stomach and breathe normally to the abdomen. (Figure 3–110(b)) When you begin to feel uncomfortable, using the hands to steady and hold the chair that the head and shoulders are on, lower the buttocks and feet to the floor. Sit up and place the tongue on the roof of the mouth and let the energy flow in the Microcosmic Orbit. (Figure 3–110(c)) Do not stand up right away as you may feel dizzy.

(5) After you have practiced for two to four weeks, you can start, very carefully, to move the chairs further apart so that only the neck

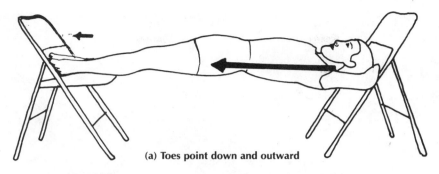

(a) Toes point down and outward

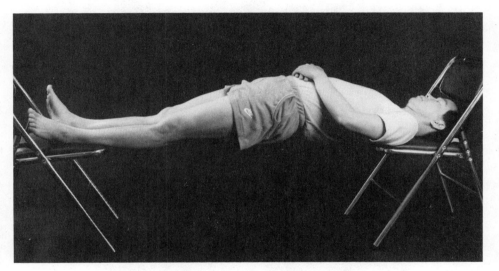

(b) Place the palms on the navel and breathe normally.

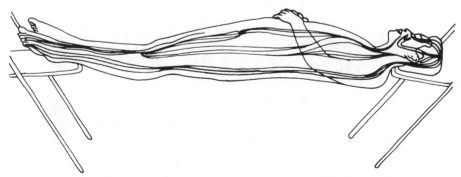

(c) The small toes' meridians running up the front and back hold the body rigid as you let the energy flow through the Microcosmic Orbit

FIGURE 3-110

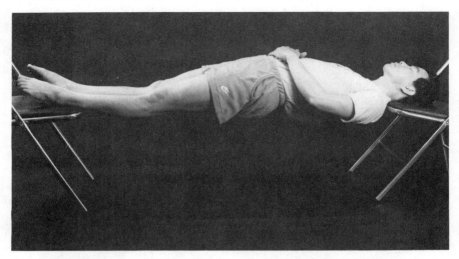

(d) Once you are well-trained, you can move the chairs further apart so that only the neck, head and heels are resting on the chairs

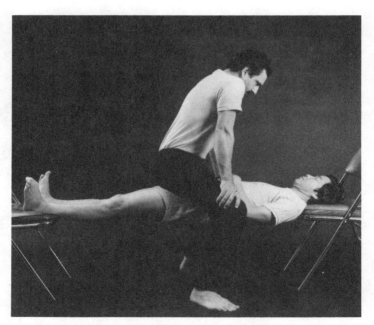

(e) In the advanced practice of the Iron Bar, you can add weight and still maintain the position

FIGURE 3-110

and head are on the end of the other chair. (Figure 3–110(d)) Do not rest the head only as this can hurt your neck.

This is a very strenuous exercise for the back. Do not attempt to move the chairs further apart unless you feel very strong. You can step up training by supporting a weight on the abdomen. Again, work gradually. Eventually you will be able to support 30 pounds or more of weight. (Figure 3–110(e))

b. Iron Bar Rooting

Have your partner place one hand under your back for support in case you should begin to fall. With the other hand, your partner presses down on your abdomen slowly and gently, increasing pressure gradually.

This exercise strengthens the lower back in the lumbar region and the psoas muscle.

10. Summary of the Iron Bar

a. Put two chairs across from one another at a distance that will allow you to:

(1) Place the feet and lower legs on one chair with the toes pointed down and outward, away from you, to develop the most balanced alignment of force in the legs, particularly in the calves.

(2) Place both palms down on the floor behind you and the head and shoulders on the other chair.

(3) Maintain a straight back. To avoid stress in the lower spine while practicing, consciously tighten the buttocks and feel the sacrum squeeze down. This will lengthen the lower spine.

(4) Breathe normally from the abdomen.

(5) When you are ready, come down to the ground slowly.

(6) Stand up and collect the energy at the navel.

(7) Practice the Bone Breathing Process.

4. BREATH ALIGNMENT

BY TERRY GOSS*

A. Structural Alignment and Taoist Yoga

Radiant health and efficient, powerful movement patterns are attained only when the body structure conforms more closely to its inherent structural pattern. This ideal pattern is the blueprint for the "stacking" of body segments in space. The function of this more appropriate structural relationship is the unhindered flow of energy, breathing, alertness and movement.

The development and use of an aligned structure is basic to Iron Shirt practice. However, for many students it will be difficult to apply principles of alignment in their practice without first approaching structural development in its own right. That is the purpose of this chapter. The structural exercises that follow lead to actual structural reformation so that "posturing" oneself according to desirable structural principles becomes easier and more natural. For most of us, without structural change "good" posture will remain alien to our being. Without intentional practice of "good" posture, particularly in the beginning, structural reintegration cannot proceed smoothly.

The anatomical relationships of the entire body are created in these structural exercises, whether moving or stationary. In structural development, it is important to conceptually understand what appropriate alignment means. Application of correct structural patterns during your practice of Iron Shirt movements will reveal their meaning and greatly speed up the process of body development. Remember that these relationships of one body part to another represent an ideal pattern. The more you practice these exercises and apply their principles in daily life, the more closely your own structure will approach the ideal in an increasingly effortless way. There should never be a sense of strain or unpleasantness in trying to "fit" the structural

*Terry Goss is a Nutrition Counselor, a Movement Educator and Yoga Instructor

220

ideal. For most people, simply a month of practice and application will lead to a profound improvement in structural health.

In the beginning of your application of these principles to daily life, there will inevitably be occasional feelings of unnaturalness. This will occur as you choose new patterns of body use which are opposed to previous distorted patterns that have become habitual. This sense of "posturing" in an artificial way will rapidly decrease with time, if you are practicing diligently. You will then experience ease and nat- uralness in body usage that allows you to respond in any direction with an appropriate amount of force. The principle of automatically applying appropriate force is at the heart of martial arts. In order for this full movement potential to be possible, the body must sponta- neously return to its "center" of relaxed alignment after movement. This is the relaxed "idling" position that is most unblocked and en- ergetically economical, and out of which movement flows.

Inanimate objects are completely dominated by the pull of gravity. Plants maintain their uprightness by the rigidity of their cell walls. Animals automatically resist the pull of gravity by normally remaining on a large base created by four legs, or two legs and a strong tail. The upright human being, on the other hand, is a unique expression of its evolving self-awareness. The full and intentional expression of stand- ing upright further develops the human spirit. Likewise, the more de- veloped human spirit naturally manifests a greater upright stance. All esoteric traditions that work with energy understand the signifiance of this fully developed upright human form. This is particularly true of the Taoist tradition.

B. Applying Structural Alignment Principles to Iron Shirt Chi Kung Practice

Diligent practice of Iron Shirt Chi Kung will lead to an increased flexibility and range of motion of the spine and other joints. As the body becomes more open, it is important to understand and apply the principles of healthy structural alignment in daily life. Since many of us have come from a background of structural randomness and distortion, it is necessary to learn what to do with our various body segments as our body becomes open and capable of new, more appropriate alignment. In effect, we must learn how best to "wear the body".

The very center of our physical structure is the spine and its foundation, the pelvis. Encased within the spine and cranium is the Central Nervous System, center of our conscious life. Thus, structural health of the spine is the foundation for the structural and energetic health of the rest of the body. For this reason, the basic structural exercises taught in this section focus strongly on the spine. Regular practice of these exercises will help heal any existing structural problems and tremendously enhance your Iron Shirt practice.

The structural exercises that follow: Structural Training Position Against Wall, Spinal Elongation Breathing, Door Hanging, Shoulder Widening and Backbend, develop a straighter, more elongated spine and joint spaces that are not cramped. The spine will retain its three normal curves, but these curves will not be as excessive as they are in nearly everyone. Attention to details will guarantee that your practice is safe, effective and progressive. Also, additional exercises (the Warrior Poses) are described that complement the practice of Iron Shirt Chi Kung by eliminating structural blocks in the hips and back, and by strengthening the lower body.

By applying the structural principles during your Iron Shirt practice, as well as in your daily life, you will feel the primary forces that are always acting on your structure. These two basic forces are (1) a strong downward rooting force connecting you to the earth; and, at the same time, (2) a strong upward elongating force lengthening your spine which connects you to the heavens. To attain balance and integration, both of these forces must be developed.

1. Relaxation

a. The Lower Abdomen

At the level of the navel center and the Door of Life (located behind the navel), rooting and elongating forces originate and mingle. For this to happen fully, the lower abdomen must always remain relaxed. The lower abdomen should remain soft, except when you are making a full exhalation, such as when you are very active, or practicing abdominal breathing. The rest of the time (which is most of the time), practice releasing any tension in the lower abdomen until this becomes automatic. Your breathing, digestion and elimination will improve, and the rest of your body will relax more fully.

The two central points of the body that reflect and determine your tension level in daily life are your face and lower abdomen. During your daily activities, practice smiling with the eyes and face, and keep your lower abdomen relaxed. Remember always to relax as much as possible, no matter what you are doing. You will feel much happier, your organs will work better and your energy will flow more easily.

b. The Inner Smile

While practicing these structural alignment exercises, also practice the Inner Smile. If you can maintain the Inner Smile while practicing vigorous exercises like Iron Shirt and the Warrior Poses, you will be able easily to maintain it during times of emotional challenge as well. Remember that the face is not only the primary expresser of body language, but also returns to your system the very emotions it expresses outwardly.

Intentionally develop the various details of facial alignment that accompany soft, relaxed, smiling eyes whenever you exercise, and you will gain much more energy and emotional balance from your practice.

When you practice the Inner Smile, let all of the facial muscles relax. This relaxation can be seen and felt particularly around the eyes and mouth. Feel the eyelids subtly close slightly as the area around the eyes relaxes, and the space between the eyebrows widens. Let the eyes be gently receptive to incoming visual stimuli. Feel that sights and sounds flow into their respective organs, rather than being grasped for outwardly. Allow the nostrils and sinuses to subtly widen, creating more space for the breath to enter the body. Let the outer corners of the mouth lift very gently, with the tongue up to the palate, the lips slightly touching, and the jaws just separated or barely touching. This will produce a smile like that of the Mona Lisa or Buddha. This lifting of the corners of the mouth must be effortless, and the outer result of an inner smile. (Figure 4–1(a))

If you can relax deeply enough, all of these details will take place spontaneously because they are natural aspects of healthy facial alignment in a happy, centered person. Practicing them intentionally will quickly condition them into your basic neuromuscular patterns.

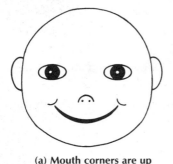

(a) Mouth corners are up

FIGURE 4-1

Inner Smile

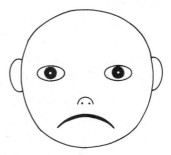

(b) Mouth corners are
down, causing the
organs to fall and
the CHI energy to
diminish

Practice the Inner Smile in this way with your eyes opened as well as closed. This will enable you to apply it at all times. A smile in the eyes and the subtle lift at the outer corners of the mouth are the most important details. Whenever you do this, it will be easy to have access to feelings of inner happiness, serenity and compassion.

Feeling the Inner Smile and relaxed facial alignment during Iron Shirt will insure that the mind remains more centered and calm, and that you are continuous and fluid in your movement. As a result, you can experience and develop the flow of CHI. (Figure 4–1(b))

c. Tight Jaw Muscles

Chronically tight jaw muscles are very common. They often distort the entire facial structure. Clenched or tightened jaws become that way for various reasons. Strong emotions that are held back from expression may produce this. On the other hand, the universal distortion of a collapsed neck in which the chin moves forward out of alignment will often cause compensations in the jaw pattern. Whatever the cause, tight jaw muscles need to be loosened up so that you can fully practice the Inner Smile and relax completely throughout the body.

Since it is difficult to relax the jaw muscles simply through intention, a cork can be useful. (Figure 4–2) This is a very beneficial exercise for people who have a lot of jaw tension, although practically anyone can benefit from trying it. Buy a simple cork stopper in a grocery or hardware store. Cut it if necessary to fit between the front teeth, thus keeping the mouth wide open. Make the width of the cork such that it is still possible to open the mouth a little farther, so that holding the cork does not result in strain. Simply place the cork in the mouth for about ten minutes every day for several weeks. As the jaw muscles stretch open, use a longer cork until you can easily use a normal sized one. This can be done while reading, driving, showering, or watching TV. Do not do this if it produces pain, if your jaws make audible sounds when they open and close, or if you have a history of jaw dislocation or other problems.

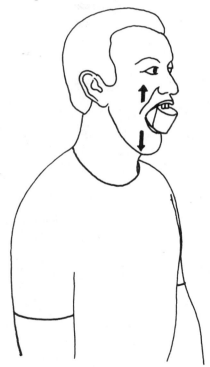

FIGURE 4-2

Practice to Stretch Tight Jaw Muscles

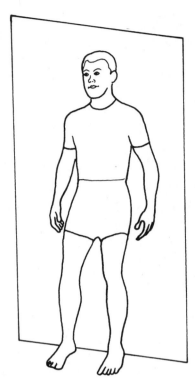

FIGURE 4-3

Structural Training Position Against Wall

2. Structural Training Position Against Wall (Figure 4–3)

Using a wall for feedback, you will be able to feel when you have a structurally aligned, elongating spine. This exercise is dependent only upon a wall or door to lean against, so it can be done anywhere as a postural recharging exercise. For those with back problems, particularly lower back pain and sciatica, it is a powerful method for decompressing the vertebrae and lessening the discomfort.

a. Lower Body

Lean against a wall with the heels approximately one to one and a half feet from the wall. Bend the knees and tuck the pelvis under so that the lower spine becomes flattened to the wall without discomfort. Work gradually to this position if there is discomfort initially. The calves will be perpendicular to the ground or slightly angled back toward the wall. You should feel that you are comfortably leaning against the wall.

b. Feet

Press the balls of the big toes firmly to the floor, then widen the feet across the balls. This will spread the toes. Now, equalize the weight on three points of each foot: the ball of the big toe, the last two toes and the middle of the heel. The toes should remain relaxed without grasping the floor with the second toes pointing straight ahead. Keep the feet aligned in this way, even if you feel pigeon-toed. Apply this same foot alignment when standing, walking or exercising.

c. Head/Neck/Upper Back

Bring as much of the upper back as flat to the wall as possible without strain, by beginning with the sacrum against the wall while holding the remainder of the spine rounded forward away from it. Now roll the spine vertebra by vertebra against the wall until you reach your limit of flexibility. Hold the head as if it is gently pushed back from the upper lip and lifted (or suspended) from its crown. Do not overdo this by tucking the chin. For many persons, the back of the head will not touch the wall. (Figure 4–4)

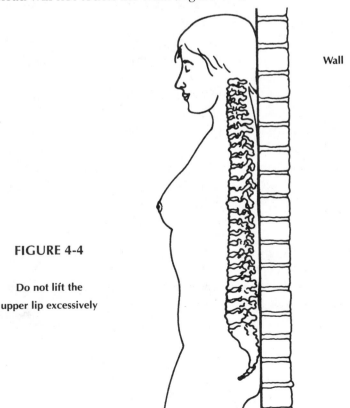

Wall

FIGURE 4-4

**Do not lift the
upper lip excessively**

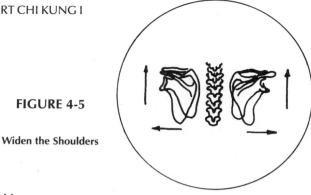

FIGURE 4-5

Widen the Shoulders

d. Shoulders

Tuck the shoulders down away from the ears and widen them out to the sides. (Figure 4–5) (See the Shoulder Widening Exercise in this Chapter.)

e. Arms/Shoulders

There are several possible arm positions:

(1) Simply let the arms hang relaxed at the sides with the palms facing into the torso. This is the most natural position and is appropriate if you are practicing around other people, at work for example, and do not want to look like you are doing an "exercise".

(2) Starting from position (1) bring the elbows back to barely touch the wall, without bringing the forearms to the wall or the shoulders back. This position helps to properly align the shoulders. As the elbows are brought back, the shoulders will naturally roll back slightly, without being pulled back excessively.

(3) Roll the left shoulder blade away from the wall until only the inner edge of the left shoulder blade is touching the wall. Now, roll the rest of the left shoulder blade back to touch the wall. Repeat on the right side, then bring the arms to position (1) or (2). This position strongly stretches the shoulders out to either side, and thus widens the upper back and chest simultaneously. This stretch is good preparation for the Iron Shirt exercises which require scapulae power.

Do not attempt positions (2) or (3) unless they can be done without strain.

f. Stretching the Lower Spine

For additional stretch in the lower back, bend the knees and sink down lower on the wall. Then, keeping the sacrum in firm contact with the wall, slowly straighten the knees back to the original position. For even more stretch, place the hands around the hips and push down while you straighten back to the original position. This will strongly lengthen the lower spine. Do not attempt this until the lower back can be brought to the wall without discomfort. This is most effective when practiced against a wall that is not completely smooth. This extra stretch is particularly valuable for anyone with lower back pain or sciatica.

g. Spinal Elongation Breathing

Simply standing in the Structural Training Position Against Wall will help to decompress and straighten the spine. It is not necessary to do special breathing in order to derive benefit from this position. The goal is not to have a straight spine, but a straightening spine. The wall gives you feedback when your spine is in a more straightened alignment.

In a structurally balanced body, breathing causes a natural elongation of the spine. This occurs to the greatest degree when the chest is filled during inhalation. The lifting and widening of the ribs causes the vertebrae to separate from each other and the spine to lengthen. Practice of deep chest breathing in this position and in Door Hanging leads to a conditioning of this natural breathing/alignment relationship. (Figure 4–6) Once you have developed this spinal elongation, it

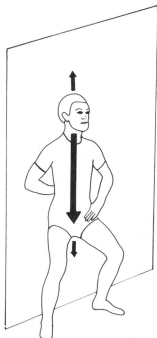

FIGURE 4-6

**Stretching the Spine
and Spinal Elongation
Breathing**

229

will occur even in the more relaxed, daily-life breathing that is primarily abdominal. This opening and closing of the spine with breathing is an integral part of the normal body mechanism that pumps blood, CHI and cerebrospinal fluid around the central nervous system.

3. How to Practice Spinal Elongation Breathing

a. Inhalation

To enhance the effects of the Structural Training Position Against Wall and the use of the breath, first fully exhale. Then, inhale slowly and deeply through the nose, directing the breath up into the chest. The abdomen should remain in and not protrude. As you do this, visualize and feel the spine lengthen. This will happen automatically if you stay relaxed. Do not try too hard. Once you feel spinal elongation, you can refine this sense further by feeling a wave of elongation starting at the base of the spine, traveling upwards as you inhale.

b. Exhalation

As you exhale, continue to feel yourself lengthening upwards, rather than collapsing back completely. You will feel the structural muscles around the spine "take over". The lengthening upwards that occurs with exhalation is more subtle than that which occurs with inhalation, and is really a wave of support that prevents excessive collapse. This wave of support begins at the head, and travels downwards as you exhale.

c. Abdominal Tightening

Because of structural blockage in the chest, it may be necessary at first to tighten the abdominal muscles in order to direct the breath up into the chest. Do this if necessary. Otherwise the abdomen will protrude as you inhale with very little chest expansion. Over time, gradually use less and less force to hold the abdomen in while inhaling, until you can breathe into the chest without either intentional abdominal contraction or unintentional abdominal protrusion.

d. Daily Life Breathing

Breathing into the chest in this way is meant as an exercise to release structural blockage in the chest and lengthen the spine fully.

After you have finished practicing, forget about your breathing and let it flow naturally. Natural breathing begins in the abdomen and only expands the chest when you are very active and, thus, breathing very fully. Do not maintain this type of full chest breathing constantly in daily life or you may cause energy to congest in the chest and head.

4. Head/Neck Alignment as the Basis for Spinal Elongation and Upright Structure

Spinal Elongation breathing cannot lengthen the spine unless the head is held as if it is pushed back from the upper lip and lifted from its crown without strain. (Figure 4–7) If the chin moves slightly forward and up, the neck collapses and the entire upper body will be collapsed and distorted. Then the spine will curve excessively and no

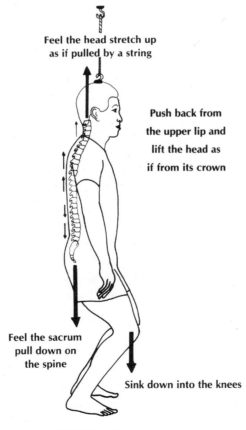

Feel the head stretch up
as if pulled by a string

Push back from
the upper lip and
lift the head as
if from its crown

Feel the sacrum
pull down on
the spine

Sink down into the knees

FIGURE 4-7

Proper alignment of the head and neck is the basis for
effective spinal elongation and an upright structure

type of deep, free breathing is possible. Even the wind pipe itself becomes constricted. This is the condition of most people's necks. For this reason, it is rare to find people in our culture who do not have chronic misalignment of the neck vertebrae.

The feeling that the head is suspended from its crown and gently pushed back from the upper lip without strain should be applied at all times. It is the foundation for an erect upper body and free breathing. Appropriate alignment of the head and neck insures a healthy communication between the body and head. Thus, awareness spreads more fully to the whole body. In a higher meditation formula of the Healing Tao System called Lesser Enlightenment of the Kan and Li, one learns to observe oneself with the inner I/eye. In the body structure, conscious alignment of the head and neck without strain is the foundation for a greater awareness that results from self-observation and self-awareness. In the practice of Hatha Yoga, elongation of the back of the neck that results from head/neck alignment is called "the root of watchfulness," or "the root of mindfulness".

Even after balanced structural alignment becomes easy and natural, a very subtle intention to maintain head/neck alignment may be necessary. This slight lifting and moving back of the head is the single most important factor in erecting the entire body. The actual elongation and shifting back of the head is often only a very small change. Without it, however, the chest, upper back and entire spine cannot come into alignment. This importance is due to the fact that the neck and head are the upper end of the column that we wish to lift. The importance of this one factor of neck and head alignment cannot be overstressed. Whole body integration is not possible without it.

It is useful to be familiar with the feeling of neck collapse that afflicts nearly everyone. After aligning the body, let the chin move forward and up, and thus out of alignment. Notice how the back of the neck shortens, the throat closes, the sternum sinks, the chest closes, the upper back arches excessively, the shoulders roll forward, breathing is restricted, and spinal elongation becomes impossible. Then practice a Spinal Elongation breath as the head is once again placed appropriately and feel the sense of full openness that accompanies it throughout the body.

Greater self-awareness, full uprightness of the trunk, and unstrained alignment of the head and neck are integrally related. The interplay of these three factors is particularly evident in Iron Shirt. The intention required to maintain head/neck alignment and the other aspects of fully aligned structure is an expression of the autonomous will of a self-aware being. Likewise, relaxed practice of fully aligning oneself develops this autonomous will in a beneficial way.

5. Door Hanging

Developing a straighter, more elongated spine is the purpose of both the Door Hanging Position and the Structural Training Position Against Wall. In Door Hanging, however, the arms are held over the head, which puts a traction on the spine and greatly increases spinal lengthening. (Figure 4–8) Daily practice of Door Hanging for even a

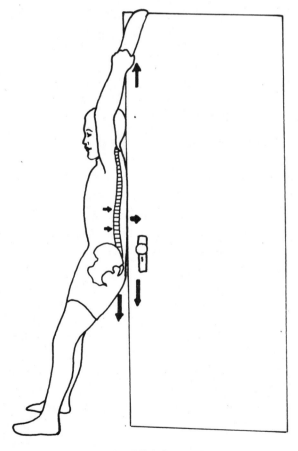

FIGURE 4-8

Door Hanging

few weeks will lead to better posture, a more flexible spine, reduction of chronic back stress and a heightened awareness of natural structural alignment. Door Hanging will also help you to be aware of and control your psoas muscles, which are very important in many Healing Tao practices.

a. Basic Position

Roll up a towel and place it over the top of a door. Lean against the narrow edge of the door, bringing the spine as flat to the edge as possible without discomfort. Follow all position details for Structural Training Position Against Wall, except those for the arms.

b. Lower Ribs/Middle Back

Maintain your attention at the lower ribs, and the middle and lower spine. Bring the arms overhead without letting the spine come away from the edge of the door. Feel that you are tucking the lower ribs in as the arms are brought overhead.

c. Hands/Arms/Shoulders

Grasp the towel fairly high, but with the elbows at least a little bent. Continue strongly to pull the shoulders down, and widen them to the sides. Do not hang from the towel. All of the body weight is still on the legs.

d. Shoulder Strain

If the shoulders are strained in this position, hold the towel lower to decrease the shoulder stretch. If necessary, the elbows may be only shoulder height or even lower. If a towel is not long enough for this, use a thick rope. Gradually you will be able to hold the towel higher, as your shoulder joints become more flexible. The first position of the Backbend exercise will also help limber your shoulder joints.

e. Breathing/Full Spinal Elongation

While maintaining this position, practice breathing up into the chest, as in Spinal Elongation breathing or the Structural Training Position Against Wall exercises described above. Along with the traction of the arms overhead, filling the chest during inhalation will result in tremendous spinal elongation. It will not take much practice to feel your spine start to lengthen. As you feel this start to happen, after every five breaths or so, bring the pelvis and the lower and middle spine a few inches away from the door edge. This allows the length-ened upper spine to lengthen further down the door. Again bring the spine and pelvis back to the door edge and continue practicing.

f. Time

If possible, practice from one to three minutes or longer. Do not continue if discomfort begins. Straining will not open your spine up faster; it will add more tightness. Regular practice and respecting your own limits will inevitably lead to very rapid spinal elongation and realignment.

g. Leaving the Position

To leave the Door Hanging position, walk the feet back toward the door and come straight up. Do not come up by pushing the pelvis away from the door first.

h. Full Hanging

If you are completely comfortable with steps a through g, you can end by letting your full weight hang from the towel. Gradually bend the knees and slide down the door edge until the arms are straight and holding you up entirely. All other details of practice are the same. Hold this for as long as comfortable, which may only be a few seconds, then come up. Be sure to continue stabilizing the shoulders by feeling them pull down and widen to the sides. Practice of Full Hanging is very strengthening and produces tremendous spinal extension, but must not be attempted if it causes strain.

6. The Psoas Muscles

a. Feeling and Using the Psoas Muscles

Once you feel comfortable with the details of Door Hanging, con-sciously relax the abdominal wall while you practice. As you soften the abdominal muscles, relax and straighten the spine against the door edge. You will be able to feel a sensation of "pulling in and up" deep inside behind the front lower ribs. This is the left and right psoas muscles working. (Figure 4–9)

Feel this same sensation of pulling in and up deep inside behind the front lower ribs when you walk and sit. This will keep your lower spine lengthened and comfortable without needing to "suck in your

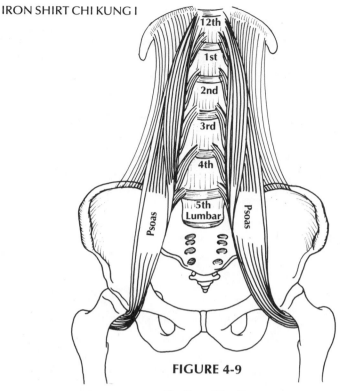

FIGURE 4-9

The Psoas Muscles

gut". Pulling in the abdomen to flatten the belly or straighten the lower
spine will hamper your energy flow and organ function. However,
working the psoas properly will not only align the lower spine, but
will also flatten the belly without tightening it.

When you carry the head as if gently pushed back from the upper
lip and suspended from its crown, the tendency is to let the lower
ribs push forward. To prevent this, feel that you are keeping the lower
ribs tucked back slightly. Remember to keep the lower ribs tucked
back from inside, not from tightening the abdomen. This will put you
in touch with the psoas alignment. You are not actually sinking the
lower ribs back, for this would cause you to slouch. You are instead
keeping them in a straight line with the abdomen below and the chest
above. Feeling the tucking sensation will stabilze the mid-torso, and
allow the whole spine to lengthen equally. The feeling, once it is developed, is that there is a subtle pulling back and up deep inside at

the lower rib area. Experience this first in Door Hanging, then apply it at all times. Like all structural improvement, intention is required initially. Gradually it will become automatic.

Door Hanging is the key to developing this psoas feeling. If the spine remains on the door and the abdomen is soft, then you need only relax and gradually sense what is already happening inside. It also helps to have a good mental picture of the anatomy involved.

Once you have developed this psoas feeling, you will find how important it is in all of the Healing Tao practices. During your practice of Iron Shirt, when you are using reverse breathing to pack the abdomen, slightly increase the psoas work of pulling in and up behind the front lower ribs. This will allow you to pack even more fully, but without tightening the abdominal wall to do it. Gradually, you will be able to pack very powerfully, with very little abdominal tension at all. When you thrust back at T–11 to pack the lower back, apply the psoas work very strongly and you will be able to focus your force to the T–11 area much more directly.

b. The Psoas Muscles and the Six Healing Sounds

The relationship between the psoas alignment and the lower rib area can be felt very well when practicing the Six Healing Sounds. (For detailed information on the Six Healing Sounds, see the book, *Taoist Ways to Transform Stress into Vitality.*) Remember to keep the lower rib area back using the psoas muscles, not by tightening the abdomen. For the Lung, Liver and Heart Sounds, be sure to keep the lower ribs held in. Then, while exhaling and making the unvoiced sound, you can put pressure within each organ more effectively. While exhaling, continuously increase the pressure to the particular organ area. At this point you will feel that you are "wringing out" the stale energy from each organ with this pressure.

Using the correct psoas alignment as you inhale will allow you to direct the fresh energy from your breath directly into the organ area more easily. When doing the Liver Sound, tilt to the right and slightly forward. Do this tilting from the lower rib area. This will increase the pressure you can apply to the liver. For the Heart Sound, tilt to the left and slightly forward, and stretch the heart meridian by stretching the little finger. For the Lung Sound, stretch the lung meridian by stretching the thumb.

For the Kidney and Spleen Sounds, the lower ribs should sink back so that you can apply pressure in each organ. When the lower ribs sink back, you are really accentuating the psoas stretch. Using the psoas muscles corectly will improve your practice of the Six Healing Sounds. By simply practicing the Six Healing Sounds you will become aware of the psoas alignment, particularly when the arms are over-head.

7. Standing Pelvic Alignment

Balanced alignment of the psoas muscles is also essential for correct leg movement and pelvic alignment. However the feet are placed, be sure that the pelvis is not tilted back or pushed to one side. The knees should remain at least slightly bent, and the arches of the feet lifted by distributing the weight equally on the three corners of each foot.

If the pelvis is askew or the knees locked back, there is stress in the lower back and knees and integration between the lower and upper halves of the body becomes impossible. For most people, maintaining structural alignment in the lower body while "standing around" requires more intention than aligning the upper body, though it is also dependent on upper body alignment. This is due to weakness in the legs and buttocks. Maintaining an aligned stance during daily life will do a great deal to strengthen the lower body, improve energetic flow, and heal lower back problems.

8. Sitting Posture

When you sit erectly for meditation, be sure that the "sitting bones" of the pelvis are directed straight down into the chair seat. Tucking the chin slightly will align your spine and give a gentle pull to the spinal cord. Then energy will flow more easily into the back portion of the Microcosmic Orbit. If you find that placing your hands in your lap causes your shoulders to roll forward or your upper back to become uncomfortable, place your hands on a thin cushion or folded blanket in your lap to alleviate this. When your CHI flow is strong, this will no longer be a problem. (Figure 4–10)

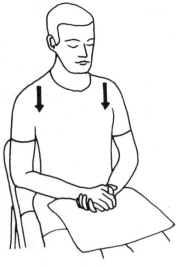

FIGURE 4-10

Practice the Microcosmic Orbit while in the sitting position

9. Shoulder Widening Exercise

The Shoulder Widening exercise develops natural alignment of the shoulders by widening the shoulder blades out to the sides, rather than rolling them forward or pulling them back. In all body segments, healthy alignment leads to an increase of space. If the shoulders are pulled back, then the width of the upper back is decreased and the upper spine is compressed. If the shoulders are rolled forward, the chest collapses and its width is decreased. However, if the shoulders are dropped down and widened out to the sides, then there is an equal opening of space across both the front and back of the upper torso.

In several of the Iron Shirt exercises, flexibility and control is developed by widening the shoulder blades out to the sides. One feels the chest sink in, but not collapse, and the shoulders drop down. This movement makes the necessary connection to the rib cage, which will permit the CHI energy to flow, thus giving the practitioner scapulae power. Remember to let the shoulders return to a natural "idling" position of dropped and widened out to the sides after your Iron Shirt practice. Do not permit them to roll forward at all so that there will be no significant loss of potential scapulae power.

a. Position for Practice

You can practice while sitting, standing, or in the Structural Alignment Position Against Wall. Be sure that the spine is erect. Aligned placement of the shoulders must begin with an erect neck/head and an erect upper back/chest.

b. Hands/Arms/Applying Force

Hold each wrist with the opposite hand. Keep the arm down low near the torso rather than lifted. Gently, but firmly, pull the elbows out to the sides without letting go of the hands. Be sure the shoulders are kept consciously dropped. Let the force at the elbows be reflected up to the shoulder joints which will increase the sense of widening at the shoulders. This is a subtle feeling, but can very definitely be felt. (Figure 4–11)

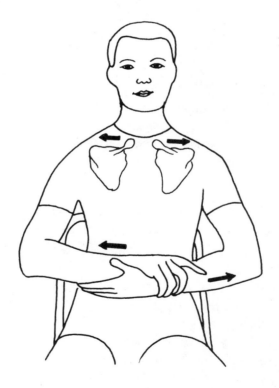

FIGURE 4-11

Shoulder Widening Exercise

c. Releasing the Force

Slowly release the pulling out of the elbows and the active dropping and widening of the shoulders. Maintain the same dropped and widened position of the shoulders which are now in a relaxed state with the arms hanging loosely at your sides.

d. Rolled-Forward Shoulders

If your shoulders are usually rolled forward, you will also need to roll them back simultaneously while performing this exercise. Be sure not to roll them back so far that the shoulder blades begin to move toward each other.

e. Practicing without Holding the Wrists

While practicing this exercise, feel which muscles are doing the work of active shoulder alignment. Muscles in both the chest and back will be working. Then, after mastering a through d above, begin to practice actively aligning the shoulders while the arms remain at your sides. You will be able to align the entire upper body easily and quickly whenever you wish. Be sure to maintain the dropping and widening of the shoulders, even when you raise the arms above shoulder height. This stabilizes the shoulders and makes arm movement steadier and more grounded while lessening the build-up of tension in the shoulders and neck.

10. Backbend

The Backbend stretches the upper back and spine opposite to the normal direction of its curve. This helps lessen the often excessive forward curve of the upper back, limbers the shoulder joints, and opens the chest.

The Backbend is the most important stretch for a healthy upper spine and freer breathing pattern. The Backbend is also very good preparation for the Iron Bridge.

a. Back Position

Roll up a blanket tightly and place it on the floor. Lie over the blanket so that it is just below the top of the shoulders. Lengthen the spine by tucking the pelvis forward to straighten the lower spine, and tuck

241

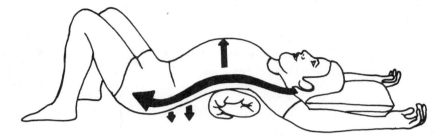

FIGURE 4-12

Position of Back During Backbend

the chin in to lengthen the back of the neck. If there is any discomfort in the back, the blanket is too high. (Figure 4–12)

b. Neck Support

If there is any discomfort in the neck after tucking in the chin and elongating the back of the neck, it is essential to place the head on another blanket or cushion. This extra neck support should be lower than the one under your back, but high enough to eliminate any neck strain and allow you to feel that the back of the neck is lengthening.

As you practice over time and gradually increase the height of the rolled-up blanket, it may be necessary to use a neck support, even though one was not needed when you used a lower rolled-up blanket. This is particularly true in the first position when the blanket is just below the top of the shoulders.

c. Arms

Slowly bring the arms back to rest on the floor above the head with the elbows well bent. Only do this if it can be done without strain. If bringing the arms back causes discomfort, they can remain at the sides, or be brought back only so far as produces stretch without strain. If brought back only part way, the arms can either be held there or placed on a cushion, piece of furniture or other prop. As the shoulder joints become more limber, the arms can be brought lower. As the arms are brought back, be sure to continue keeping the shoulder blades dropped and widened.

d. Breathing

While relaxing in this Backbend posture, breathe deeply and slowly, directing the breath to fill the chest rather than expand the abdomen. This greatly increases the stretch of the spine and chest. If necessary, hold the abdomen in while inhaling so that chest expansion can occur. It may seem very difficult initially to breathe up into the chest while practicing the Backbend, but practice will be rewarded by a great deal of structural opening in the chest and upper back.

e. Several Positions for Blanket

In order to limber the whole upper spine and shoulder joints, practice the Backbend in each of the following positions. Do not practice with the blanket below the sternum.

First position: The blanket is just under the tops of the shoulders. Second position: The blanket is under the middle of the chest. Third position: The blanket is under the bottom of the sternum.

f. Time/Resting Between Positions

Remain in each position for several minutes or more if you are comfortable. Most people find the Backbend very pleasant from the beginning: similar to getting a back massage. If the Backbend is initially a difficult stretch for you, leave the position and rest before continuing to the next position. Once the Backbend is easy and pleasant, you can shift from first to second to third positions on the blanket without coming up first.

g. Leaving the Position

To get up after the Backbend, use your hand to lift your head to a chin-on-chest position, then roll off the blanket to one side before sitting up. This will prevent strain on the neck or back.

h. Forward Bend

Ideally, bend over forward and relax after the Backbend and upon completion of the Iron Bridge. The knees should be at least slightly bent. If the knees are locked back, they will be strained. If you want to stretch farther forward, do not increase the forward curvature of the upper spine in doing so. Stretch forward by letting the hamstring muscles at the backs of the thighs lengthen. If you are stretching forward vigorously, or are not very limber, bend the knees much more while stretching so that you can lay the whole abdomen firmly on the thighs. Then, test your flexibility by slightly straightening the knees while keeping the abdomen on the thighs. Practicing in this way will guarantee that you are only stretching the lower spine and hamstrings, and not arching the upper spine.

i. Increasing the Height of the Blanket

As the upper back becomes more limber, continue to increase the height of the rolled-up blanket(s) in order to feel a strong stretch but no discomfort.

11. Warrior Poses 1 and 2

Practice of both Warrior Poses leads to great flexibility and strength in the buttocks and legs. As the strength and flexibility develop, there is structural opening and realigning in the hip/thigh/lower back area that is essential in Iron Shirt. The awareness created in the Warrior Poses develops the ability strongly to use the lower body in movement or in standing, without compressing the lower spine or neck.

a. Warrior Pose 1 (Figure 4–13(a) and (b))

(1) Feet

Stand with the left foot straight ahead and the right foot turned in 45 degrees. A line through the middle of the left heel should intersect the middle of the arch of the right foot. Throughout the exercise, keep equal weight on the three points of each foot. The distance between the two feet should be as wide as possible without losing the indicated alignment for the lower back and back leg.

(2) Pelvis/Lower Back

Start with both legs straight at the knees. Strongly turn the pelvis under, so that the lower back is straight. This will require strong buttocks work. It is absolutely essential that the lower back remains in this straightened position throughout the exercise. If the feet are too far apart, this will be impossible.

(3) Spinal Extension

After flattening the lower spine, extend upward through the whole spine. Hold the head as if it is gently pushed back from the upper lip and lifted from its crown. Be sure that the front lower ribs remain in.

244

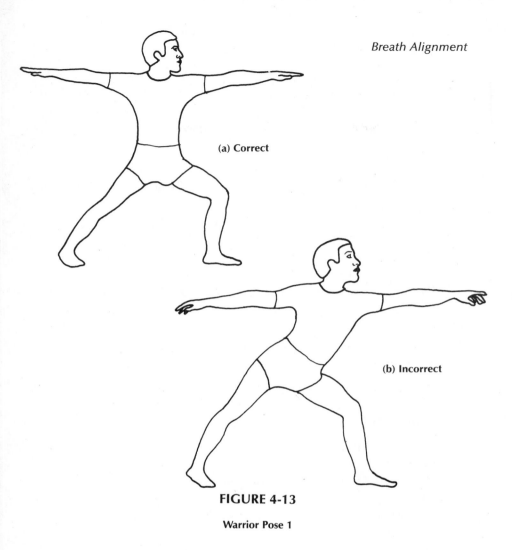

(a) Correct

(b) Incorrect

FIGURE 4-13

Warrior Pose 1

Do not permit the lower rib area to push forward. This is particularly true in these Warrior Poses, and more so in Warrior Pose 2 than in Warrior Pose 1. Maintain a full extension of the spine throughout the exercise.

(4) Moving Into the Full Pose

Now exhale and bend the left (front) leg, until the left knee is directly over the left ankle, keeping the right (back) leg as straight as possible. Do not let the left knee move to the right as it comes forward. This would prevent the groin from opening. The knee must remain exactly over the ankle.

(5) Distance Between Feet

If the feet are too far apart, you will not be able to bend the left knee all the way over the left ankle without arching the lower spine and/or bending the back leg a lot at the knee.

(6) Back Leg

It is all right to let the back leg bend a little to keep the lower spine straight. As you are holding the position, gradually straighten the back leg more at the knee until you reach your limit. Do not straighten it to the point where your lower spine begins to arch.

(7) Time Breathing/Leaving the Pose

Maintain this position for one to two minutes, breathing slowly and deeply up into the chest to elongate the spine. Breathe continuously without any pause. Come out of the position while exhaling by first straightening the front leg. Then, turning both feet parallel to each other, place them together. Repeat for an equal time on the opposite side. (Simply reverse left and right when following the instructions).

b. Warrior Pose 2 (Figure 4–14(a) and (b))

(1) Feet

Stand with both feet facing straight ahead, the right foot several feet behind the left foot and several inches to the right. Lift the heel of the right foot off the floor. Throughout the exercise, keep equal weight on the three points of the left (front) foot and equal weight across the balls of the right (back) foot. The distance between the two feet should be as wide as possible without losing the indicated alignment for the lower back and back leg.

(2) Pelvis/Lower Back

Turn the pelvis so that the pelvis and whole torso is square with the front thigh. The navel will then be pointing exactly in the direction of the front foot. Begin with both knees straight. Strongly turn the pelvis under, so that the lower back is straight. It is absolutely essential that the lower back remains unarched throughout the exercise. If the feet are too far apart, this will be impossible.

Instructions (3) through (7) for Warrior Pose 2 are identical to Warrior Pose 1.

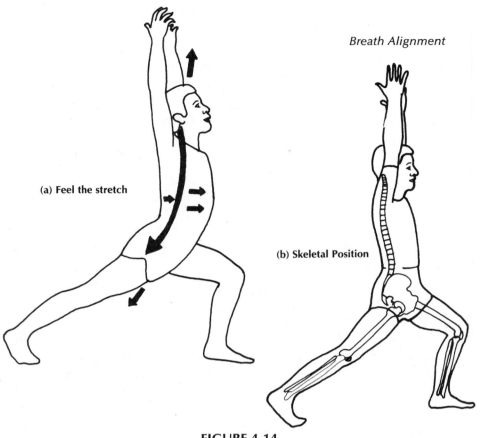

(a) Feel the stretch

(b) Skeletal Position

FIGURE 4-14

Warrior Pose 2

(8) Arms Position When Warrior Pose 2 Is Developed

When your practice has become familiar and strong, add the following arms position. Extend both arms straight up, while keeping the shoulder blades dropped and widened. The palms face each other. Pay particular attention not to let the lower rib area extend forward as the arms are extended upward.

(9) Arms Position

Because this is a very strengthening exercise, it requires strong concentration and strong (but not stressful) exertion to maintain the straight lower spine and straightening back leg. When first learning either Warrior Pose, it is usually best to use the arms to aid pelvic alignment. One hand pushes the sacrum down and forward from the back, while the other hand pushes in and slightly up at the lower ribs

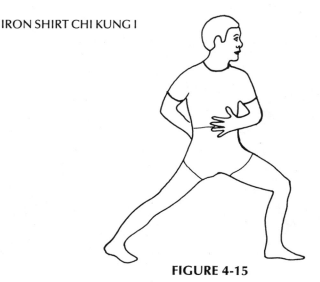

FIGURE 4-15

Arm Position for Beginners

from the front. (Figure 4–15) This helps greatly in keeping the spine straight, and you can keep all of your concentration on the lower body exertion.

(10) Further Details Of Practice

If practiced two or three times per week, strength will develop rapidly and flexibility slowly, but surely. As flexibility increases, the feet can be held farther apart from each other until finally the front thigh will be parallel to the floor while the other details of the form are maintained. This final position requires tremendous flexibility and strength. Most people will not achieve this for a long time. Just remember that an arched lower back or well-bent back knee means the feet are too far apart. It is a good idea to check your lower back in a mirror when first learning. You may be quite suprised how close the feet have to be to practice properly.

(11) Arms Position When Warrior Pose 1 Is Developed

When your practice has become familiar and strong, add the following arms position. Extend both arms strongly at shoulder height directly to the front and back. Let the eyes gaze at the tip of the second finger of the forward arm. Keep the shoulders pulled down, rather than hunched. Extend from the fingertips through each joint to the shoulder blades.

5. BODY CONSTRUCTION AND IRON SHIRT

This chapter is concerned with the construction of fasciae and their structural interrelationship with bones, muscles, and tendons. Further, instruction on the muscle tendon meridians (or acupuncture routes) of the body increases an awareness of the body's construction, which awareness is vital to the work at hand: the creation and storage of CHI energy and its circulation throughout the body. Dr. Michael Posner, a practicing Chiropractor, provides an introduction to this chapter by discussing the major keys to good health through an understanding of body structure. Learn as much as you can about the way that you are constructed because it will speed your progress. Knowing what makes you tick and how you are put together is very important in putting you in contact with yourself through Iron Shirt Chi Kung.

I. IRON SHIRT AND CHIROPRACTIC, BY DR. MICHAEL POSNER

In all health professions nowadays, one thing that is commonly considered detrimental to our health is the phenomenon of stress. Various methodologies and theories have emerged that aim to help minimize the amount of stress one has to cope with. I wish to discuss the unavoidable stress of gravity on a body's structure when in an upright position, some health implications, and how, through proper alignment of bone structure, we can efficiently minimize stress and increase good health.

As gravitational forces act upon our bodies when we are upright, various groups of musculature work so that we can stay erect. To resist gravity, these muscles must exert a certain amount of energy. These anti-gravity muscles help to stabilize the bone structure in such a way that movement is possible in an upright position. The

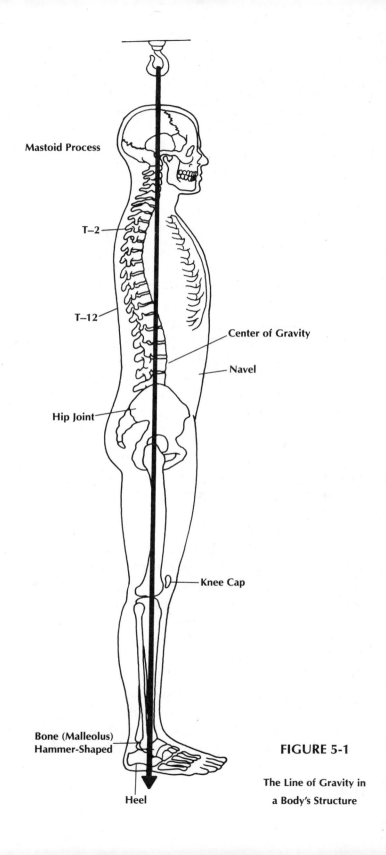

Mastoid Process

T–2

T–12

Center of Gravity

Navel

Hip Joint

Knee Cap

**Bone (Malleolus)
Hammer-Shaped**

Heel

FIGURE 5-1

The Line of Gravity in
a Body's Structure

success that a person has in meeting the constant stress of gravity may have a subtle yet profound influence on his or her quality of health, performance and emotional states.

At this point, it is necessary to understand some basic concepts such as "line of gravity" and "center of gravity" as they relate to our bodies' structures. The line of gravity, viewed laterally (Figure 5–1), anteriorly and posteriorly, falls from above downward through the earlobe, slightly behind the mastoral process (or the attachment of muscles behind the ear of the temporal bone, the bone located at the side of the head which contains the organ of hearing), through the odontoral process (a toothlike projection from the body of the axis or second vertebra of the neck upon which the first cervical vertebra rotates), through the middle of the shoulder joint, touches the mid-point of the frontal borders of T–2 and T–12, then falls just slightly outside to the sacrum, slightly behind the axis, or support, of the hip joint, slightly behind to the patella (or kneecap), crosses in front to the middle malleolus (the hammer-shaped bone on each side of the ankle) and through the outer bone of the ankle to fall between the heel and metatarsal heads. When viewed from the back, the line of gravity passes through the occipital bone (or the lower back part of the skull), C–7 and L–5, the coccyx (or lower end of the spine) and pubic cartilage (or supporting tissue of the pubic bones) and bisects the knees and ankles.

As gravity acts on all parts of the body, one's entire weight can be considered as concentrated at a point where the gravitational pull on one side of the body is equal to the pull on the other side. This point is the body's center of gravity. Generally speaking, the center of gravity is located in a region directly in front of, and about one and a half inches above and below, the level of the navel. Its location varies according to body type, age, sex, attitude, breathing patterns, stress level, or abnormal neuromusculoskeletal disorders.

The most economical use of energy in the standing position occurs when the vertical line of gravity falls through a column of supporting bone in alignment. If weight bearing bony segments are aligned so that the gravity line passes directly through the center of each joint, the least stress is placed upon the adjacent ligaments, tendons and muscles. When this alignment is achieved, the antigravity muscles which expend much energy to resist the downward pull of gravity need not work as hard. The bones now take on a more active role in supporting our bodies in an upright posture, allowing the muscles to relax and rest, thus conserving energy and diminishing stress and tensions developed from unbalanced bone and muscle patterns.

Health potentials can be realized only when balance of structure exists so that both nerve energy and CHI flow freely.

There are many negative health effects produced when these antigravity muscles are working either too much or too little. Muscles function to move bones and, if muscles are either very tense or too flaccid, unilaterally or bilaterally, they will create a derangement in our bone structure. When a person feels knots or spasms in their muscles, this means that the muscle has gone into a state where it has a sustained contraction. A contraction means that the muscle fibers have shortened. As this occurs, bones can be pulled out of their proper alignment. When spinal vertebrae are involved in this structural imbalance, nerve roots can be irritated, thus interfering with the function of the nervous system. When the nervous system is interfered with, a multitude of health problems can arise since the nervous system is the means by which all body functions are regulated and monitored.

Health potentials are enhanced when proper communication between the brain and all body parts is maximized. Since this is the function of the nervous system, the structural integrity of our musculoskeletal system is of prime importance. Structure is said to determine function.

The chiropractic profession deals with problems of health and disease from a structural point of view, with special consideration given to structural intergrity, spinal mechanics and neurological relation.

Thus far, it has been shown how gravity interrelates with our musculoskeletal systems, and how this stress on our structure could affect our health in general. Of course, other factors such as emotions, toxins and trauma affect one's structure as well. Muscles store and harbor tension and stress from various sources, but the point is that structural imbalance is the end result and, in turn, our functionability is diminished, as well as our health.

From this standpoint, logically speaking, one must seriously consider how to go about producing optimum structural integrity in a balanced way. To do this, it is necessary to: understand the value in learning about alignment; learn the principles from a competent source; recognize one's own problems in this area; and then apply the knowledge to oneself.

As a chiropractor, I am concerned with correcting each patient's structure to allow the body's optimum function to be restored. But I can only do so much for a person and, in reality, one's health is one's own responsibility. Therefore, the necessity for everyone to learn about structure for themselves, and to recognize what is right or wrong, is essential for good health. I believe that some of the major keys to good health are proper bone alignment, muscle balance (symmetry), flexibility of joints and fasciae, proper breathing, relaxation and proper body utilization. Finally, of extreme importance, is to learn to conserve, build and store energy that is usually wasted when structural imbalance exists.

Exercise is an indispensible means to attain the above keys to health. The kind of exercise, therefore, must not be unilateral, as most sports are, and not tension producing (i.e., not in excess). Well-toned muscles and fasciae are desirable, but not too much, or not too little. Balance is, therefore, the key when choosing an exercise system. The exercise system should be one that develops the body symmetrically, reduces stress, teaches proper alignment and one that shows how to store, increase and conserve vital energy.

I am a chiropractor who sees health to a great extent dependent on symmetry or balance of body structure and so became interested in the Chinese art of Iron Shirt Chi Kung. Iron Shirt emphasizes the importance of maintaining a bone posture in such a way that the gravitational forces acting to push us down to earth can be transmitted through the bones into the earth, rather than wasting energy resisting with the muscles or putting undue stress on the joints. The Iron Shirt postures align the vertebrae in such a manner as to permit the line of gravity to pass through the center of the vertebrae. Now the force is not being resisted, but rather transmitted. The muscles, ligaments and tendons can relax instead of working to resist. Integration of all structural tissues for optimum functions is created by the Iron Shirt postures. Relaxation, proper breathing, symmetrical muscle development, tendon and ligament strengthening, as well as strengthening the bones, result from Iron Shirt practice.

Another very important concept is to learn to experience and re-create one's proper center of gravity. I say "proper" because generally one's center of gravity changes from the navel area up into the chest or higher as one confronts life situations and stresses. This interferes with normal breathing patterns which should be originating from the abdomen as well as the chest. One simply has to compare a child's breathing to the breathing of most adults, and it will become evident that adults mainly breathe from their chests with very little abdominal or diaphragmatic action. It is very important that we utilize our diaphragm when breathing since the diaphragm descends upon and massages our internal visceral organs. This action enhances circulation and blood flow as well as increased oxygen to all of our vital organs.

The increased energy, structural integrity and phenomenal health benefits gained from Iron Shirt practice, in my opinion, are outstanding. I feel that its practice can develop future health potential in a wholistic way: physically, mentally, emotionally and spiritually. When one aligns oneself with Iron Shirt practice, he also aligns himself with the harmony of the universe.

II. THE CONSTRUCTION OF FASCIAE, THE RELATIONSHIP OF FASCIAE TO BONES, MUSCLES AND TENDONS, AND ACUPUNCTURE ROUTES, OR MUSCLE TENDON MERIDIANS

A. Fasciae: Protectors of Your Vital Organs

After an ovum is fertilized it differentiates into three main systems, the ectoderm, endoderm and mesoderm. Fasciae are derived from the mesenchyme, which is a subdivision of the mesoderm.

Nuclei in the mesenchymal substance give rise to bones, ligaments, muscles and tendons. Then a more structureless system of casings, sheaths and tissue takes shape around the various centers which have been developed.

The fascia is a sheath and its function is that of support, protection, mechanical advantage, some degree of contractility and lengthening, and energizing the organs and muscles to let CHI energy flow through easily. The fascia is a type of connective tissue which is avascular (or without blood vessels), translucent and tough. It is intimately involved with muscles, encasing them and enhancing their duties by various means, which include separating them into distinct bundles, providing bonds of especially tough fibers to offer support for purposes of leverage, and allowing for lubrication by means of fluids released from the tissues of an organ or part so that these enclosed muscle groups can slide over each other. Fasciae are present throughout the body, separating, connecting, wrapping and supporting various parts of it, and finally, on a superficial level, encasing the whole body in a shimmering sheath just beneath the level of the skin.

These superficial fasciae are very resilient, due to the fact that the fibers run in a criss-cross pattern. Damage by trauma alters them, making them denser and shorter, a characteristic of scar tissue.

Since this network is present throughout the body, it might explain the mechanism of trigger points, whereby the malfunction of internal organs is evidenced as pain in small areas often quite remote from the organ involved.

This might also explain another mechanism, the one found in reflexology. Certain areas of the feet might at varying times be painful, coinciding with organs in the body.

There is another little-recognized function of fasciae: that of providing muscle tone. In fact, low blood pressure is associated with a hypotonus condition of fasciae and hypertension with a hypertoned fasciae. (This means that a condition of the fasciae exist in which a high or low pressure causes too much or a limited diffusion of solutions throughout the fasciae.) There are several types of fasciae, all built of collagen. The most widely distributed is the loose connective tissue, which is the most flexible and most elastic of all, its fibers going in all directions. It consists of protein imbedded in a liquid ground substance and is very important to water metabolism and to other fluid exchanges. Tough, fibrous tissue can be found in areas where more tensile strength is required. Here the tissue is tough and unyielding, resulting from the parallel arrangement of bundles of fibers which are also found in tendons and ligaments. Huge fascial sheets found in the body are comprised of such tissue. All variations in fasciae, however, stem from the mesoderm.

The fasciae, though avascular themselves, furnish support for blood vessels, nerve fibers and vessels of the lymphatic system and contain the nerves which convey fluid into the veins and sensory receptors which are responsive to internal stimuli from the muscles, joints and tendons. The fasciae are also responsible for maintaining the relative positions of the various organs and muscles in the body.

1. Fasciae Exist in Three Layers (Figure 5–2)

a. The Superficial or Subcutaneous Layer: The superficial layer (the layer beneath the skin) is composed of two subdivisions: (1) a layer which can contain a tremendous amount of fat in those who are overweight; and (2) the more internal area of the subcutaneous fasciae. This is the most elastic of the various fasciae, since it has to accommodate varying amounts of fat storage, swelling when there is inflammation and muscular activity and distension when the muscles are

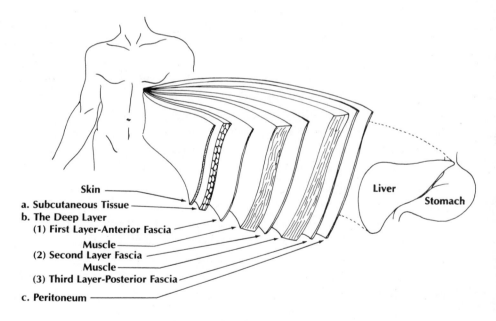

FIGURE 5-2

Fasciae Exist in Three Layers

worked. In this layer we are able to store CHI energy. As this layer of the body fills up with CHI, it is unavailable for storage of fat by the body. By practicing Iron Shirt packing, you can burn out the fat already existing in this layer.

b. The Deep Layer: The deep fasciae, which are denser and have a smooth surface, allow for a reduction in friction as one surface slides over another. The deep fasciae produce bundles of fibers in parallel arrangement, giving great tensile strength. This sort of tissue is formed around the ankles, knees, wrists and elbows where it acts as an anchor against which muscles can pull. Fasciae also act in the capacity of a nutritional storehouse, as a source of insulation and support by means of fatty content, and as a barrier to impede the entrance of foreign organisms and objects.

The deep fasciae keep muscles in their distinct shapes and positions. These fasciae, which are the densest and have the greatest tensile strength, are made up of three types. The first and outermost is the external surrounding layer. These cover large muscle groups. The intermediate membranes separate individual muscles and, finally, the internal surrounding layer covers the external surfaces of the body cavities.

c. The Subserous Layer or Peritoneum: Internal to the intermediate membrane lie the subserous fasciae, or fascial layer beneath the membranes of the body which line all of the large cavities of the body. There are two types: (1) the parietal (or cavity wall) fasciae which cover the inner surfaces of the body cavities such as the thorax or abdomen; and (2) the visceral (or internal organ) fasciae which cover the organs in those cavities such as the lungs or liver. Again the main functions are protective and supportive, as well as a means of lubrication. During irritation these serousal surfaces sometimes adhere to one another, causing great pain.

2. Iron Shirt Is Concerned with the Fasciae of the Whole Body

Iron Shirt is concerned with the fasciae of the entire body; that is to say it primarily involves the subcutaneous layer (beneath the skin) which covers the whole body. Iron Shirt is specifically concerned with the fasciae in the lumbar region, which are thicker and more fatty than ordinarily encountered. These two divisions of fasciae are joined by spindle connections, which are columnar shaped fibers between which the fat is deposited.

The lumbar fasciae are composed of three layers. The most superficial one extends out from the middle, from the spines of the lumbar verterbrae (situated near the lower rib and hip bone) and the spine of the sacrum (the bone formed by the union of five vertebrae between the lumbar and caudel, or tail) region, constituting the back part of the pelvis and sacrospinalis ligament (a muscle which extends vertically along the length of the vertebrae in that area) and also out to the sides to the intermediate layer. The intermediate layer extends from the middle of the area of the lumbar and out to the sides, where it joins with the superficial layer. These two layers envelop the muscles which hold a person erect.

The fasciae also extend upward to the lower portion of the twelfth rib and, at its lower extremity, are attached to the iliac crest (the large upper part of the pelvis) and the iliolumbar ligament, both in the small intestine area. The deepest layer envelops the quadratus lumbarum (a muscle which extends out from the area of the lumbar to join the other two layers at the sides, as previously described.) The three layers together comprise what is technically known as the "Origin of the Transverse Abdominis Aponeurosis".

The deep fasciae of the upper back are made up primarily of thoracic fasciae, which are thin coverings of the extensor muscles of the thoracic spine (vertebrae between the neck and abdomen, enclosed by ribs). Its lower border joins with the most superficial part of the tri-layer of the deep lumbar fasciae, while its upper portion combines with the cervical and trapezius fasciae. Attaching along a mid-line composed of the spines of the thoracic vertebrae, the deep fasciae of the upper back extend out to the sides following the rib angles and the fasciae of the muscles between the ribs.

The deep fasciae that enclose the rhomboids (two muscles that attach to each shoulder blade) and muscles of the posterior (or back) are considered to be separate from the thoracic fasciae, though there is no actual separation between the two.

Out to either side the axillary fasciae (covering the armpit) are to be found serving as a protective layer over the axillae which are practically devoid of muscular tissue. They also partially enclose the back and side muscles, blend in with the thoracic fasciae, and are connected to the fasciae beneath the spine. In turn, the deltoid fasciae (covering the triangular muscle of the shoulder and upper arm), at about the level of the fourth thoracic vertebra and the mid-scapular (mid-shoulder blade) line, connects with the fasciae beneath the spine and is anchored to the spine and acromion process (the shoulder blades' projections which form the points of each shoulder).

All of the various layers just mentioned combine to form the continous fascial network of the back.

The deltoid fasciae extend out from the spine at the scapulae to the clavical (or collar bone). There they merge with the pectoral fasciae (covering the breast). The deltoid fasciae also extend laterally from the shoulder into the arm where they become known as the brachial fasciae. These brachial fasciae join with the pectoral and axillary fasciae and are attached to the epicondyles of the humeri (covering the large rounded prominences associated with the shoulder joints) on the upper end of each humerus (bone of the upper arm) as well as the olecranon of each ulna (or the curved part of the ulna bone at the point of the elbow). (The ulna bone is one of two bones in the forearm and is on the same side as the pinky finger. The other forearm bone is called the radius.) The brachial fasciae are thin where they cover the biceps and thicker over the triceps.

The interbrachial fasciae join as one with the brachial fasciae and extend from the epicondyles of the humeri to the remotest ends of the radius and ulna bones.

The pectoral fasciae are thin sheaths connected to the clavicle and sternum (or breastbone) and extend to the deltoid, brachial and axillary fasciae and also the outer surrounding layer of the abdominal fascia. They also attach to the diaphragm. Beneath the pectoral fasciae lie the pectoralis major muscles. Beneath those are fascial sheaths called the clavipectoral fasciae that enclose the pectoralis minor muscles. This is found between the pectoralis minor and the thoracic body wall.

These fasciae, attached to the clavicle and enveloping the artery running beneath the clavicle, extend to the first rib, the coracoid process of the scapula (the bone that unites with the scapula to form the cavity through which the arteries of the scapula and temporal bones run) and the axillary fasciae.

The ribs comprise the foundation of the thoracic body wall and are covered exteriorally by the external intercostal fasciae (or fasciae between the ribs). This sheath, extending in the direction of the head, joins the scalene fasciae (the fasciae covering the deep muscles attached to the cervical vertebrae and first and second ribs, acting to flex or bend the neck). Extending downwards towards the lower abdomen, this sheath joins with the fasciae that separate the external and internal oblique muscles of the abdomen.

The interior surfaces of the ribs are covered by the endothoracic fasciae (surrounding the muscles within the thorax). These extend toward the head, blending with the prevertebral fasciae (covering the vetebrae which are at the beginning or top of the spinal column), while in their extension to the lower abdomen they connect to the internal surrounding layer of the abdominal wall. The subcutaneous fasciae of the abdomen are soft and pliable, increasing in tensile strength as they extend out to the sides. The highly elastic deeper portion of the subcutaneous fasciae are attached to the linea alba and the inguinal (or groin) ligament. (Alba is a white substance carried by the central nervous system.) The outer investing layer of the deep abdominal fasciae unite with the fasciae of the back and the breast. In their extension downward they connect with the fasciae lata (the external fasciae of the thighs), symphysis pubis (the junction of the two bones which join with a third to form the arch on either side of the pelvis) and the aponeurosis (the white fibrous tissue which forms the attachment of the external abdominal oblique muscles).

The surrounding internal layer unites with the deepest portion of the thoraco-lumbar fasciae, the pelvic fasciae and the fasciae of the diaphragm and are commonly referred to as the transversalis fasciae. These cover the external surface of the abdominal cavity wall, the lumbar vertebra bodies and the psoas major muscle.

The various fascial layers which have been described are integral to the cultivation of Iron Shirt as the fasciae into which we pack CHI. As previously described, this CHI will then form a protective cushion in the body which is also a storage place from which CHI can be retrieved when required.

B. *Cleansing the Marrow/Changing the Tendons*

1. "Cleansing the Bone Marrow"

The process of transforming sexual energy for storage in the brain and bone marrow, cleansing the internal organs, and restoring the organs to proper function is known as "Cleansing the Bone Marrow".

By circulating CHI in the Microcosmic Orbit and cleansing the "inner marrow" (which, as described in Chapter 1, increases the quantity of blood cells, a vital source of life-force), your system is cleansed of pollution. With the routes cleared, CHI flows freely to where it is needed and then it is said that the whole body is filled with CHI. When a person ages, the bone marrow begins to dry out and produces fewer blood cells. At that time, the body fills the empty space within the bones with fat. In order to fill the empty bones with renewed energy to revitalize the marrow to a youthful condition, we need to transfer sexual energy which can be stored in the bones while simultaneously burning out fat.

Cleansing the bone marrow, maintaining healthy organs and changing the tendons lead to a strengthening of the muscles, tendons and ligaments, a condition described as one in which the inside of the body is clean and the outside is strong. All three levels of Iron Shirt practice are involved with strengthening and rebuilding the fasciae, tendons and bone marrow.

2. "Changing the Tendons"

Using various methods, CHI can be gathered from internal organs and led out to the fasciae surrounding them whenever necessary. When sufficient CHI has been accumulated, it is guided out along the fasciae between muscle groups and finally to the tendons which themselves are included in fascial sheaths until the entire body is filled with energy.

Tendons connect muscles to bones, are stronger than muscles and last longer. Fewer cells and smaller blood supplies are required to maintain and develop the tendons. Iron Shirt is designed to strengthen and develop the tendons so that movement no longer depends strongly upon the muscles.

In Taoism your health is said to be impaired if your tendons are crooked, loose or weak. Diseased and crooked tendons will cause you to be thin and if the tendons are no longer resilient, this causes you to be easily fatigued as well. The fasciae can become restricted due to injury, resulting in scar tissue which is tougher and tends to contract and pull upon the surrounding tissues and tendons, impeding blood flow and interfering with the passage of CHI. Emotions can also be traumatic and can chronically alter your way of seeing the world and, thereby, the way in which you present yourself to the world. This is evident in many ways, most obviously by the way in which you hold yourself physically.

Fasciae and bone tendons take a longer time to grow and, when injured, take a much longer time to heal. When, however, the tendons are strong, relaxed, and long and full of strength, they are also full of large quantities of CHI and have ready access to more of it when needed. Once developed, they will be much stronger, last longer, and work harder. They will use very little nutrients and will require very little maintenence.

Some therapists have worked on loosening what has become overly restricting fascial tissue, thus often liberating emotions and memories that had created a constant drain on a person's energy reserves. Sometimes the person experiences a new lease on life by being able to function with a range of freedom of motion that he might otherwise never have known.

As previously mentioned, "Changing the Tendons" and "Cleansing the Bone Marrow" will be dealt with further in Iron Shirt II and Iron Shirt III, respectively.

C. The Harmony of Fasciae, Tendons and CHI

A Taoist would describe the body as internally consisting of the vital internal organs and the CHI energy which services them. Externally the body is comprised of bones, tendons, muscles and the fasciae which contain them. If you recall, bones are moved by the action of muscle contractions which pull on the tendons that are attached to the bones. Blood is said to move muscles and CHI to move blood.

Thus, the Taoist Master strives to create and protect the CHI and the blood. This CHI, as an electromagnetic energy, is unseen, while the muscles, tendons, bones and fasciae are quite visible. Practice consists of working both the visible and the invisible as an expression of the harmony of Yin and Yang.

To stress only internal or external development will result in disharmony and dysfunction. The organs and muscles must be vitalized by CHI, but the circulation of the CHI is augmented by having a healthy body. Strengthening muscles without cultivating CHI creates a similar imbalance which will not lead to true health or strength.

"Changing the Tendons" works with the muscles, tendons, bones and fasciae, developing both the visible (muscles, tendons, bones and fasciae) and the invisible (the flow of CHI).

The practice of loosening the tendons is comparatively easy, whereas that of utilizing the fasciae is considered to be more difficult. Iron Shirt Chi Kung is said to be the most difficult discipline of all and yet its practice, in which you learn to increase and store more CHI, truly begins with the Microcosmic Orbit. Once you have collected CHI, you can direct it as it is needed to the fasciae of any point in the body.

By a process in which you collect, conserve and reserve the energy of the vital organs (kidneys, brain, heart, liver, lungs, spleen and genitals), the polluted energy descends and exits as the clean, vital energy rises up to replace it. As you relax and collect more and more CHI, it is directed towards the tendons and fasciae until the entire body is filled with CHI energy.

The CHI flows into the fasciae, expanding and strengthening the tendons.

Again, balance or harmony is necessary. If you practice so that your fasciae are vitalized with CHI and your tendons are neglected, the fasciae will have nothing to depend on, since it is by way of the tendons that the muscles attach to the bones. On the other hand, if you work on the tendons and not the fasciae, the fasciae will not fill out and serve well as a coordinator of the muscle groups which they cover. If you exercise the tendons and the fasciae without Chi Kung to activate an energy flow, the tendons and fasciae will not "raise up" separately and will not be able to work freely. If you practice Chi Kung

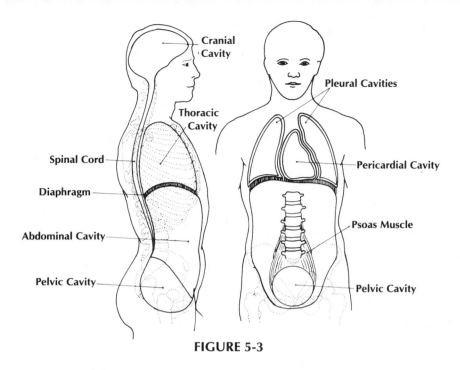

FIGURE 5-3

One of the most important reasons for practicing Iron Shirt is to fill the
cavities of the body with CHI

and not the tendon or fascia exercises, the CHI will not be able to
travel freely throughout the body and will be impeded in gaining access to all of the meridians. At the same time, the tendons will be weak
through disuse and the fasciae will be tight and restricting.

In this chapter, an overall picture is presented describing how the
muscles, fasciae and bones function together. Muscles cover other
muscles and bones and contain the various cavities which hold your
vital organs. The tendons and fasciae are joined together and the tendons connect muscles to bones. The fasciae cover muscle groups, af-
fording them the ability to do more work than they would were they
not so bound together, and add to the resilience and general tone of
the muscles as well. Since these bundles of muscles wrapped in fasciae lie outside of bones, they protect them, and since they make up
the walls of the thoracic and abdominal cavities, they protect everything within them. The most important uses of the Iron Shirt Chi
Kung are to fill the cavities of the body with CHI and to build up more
CHI pressure in the vital organs, protecting and enabling them to de-
liver instant energy. (Figure 5–3)

D. Muscle-Tendon Meridians

There are 12 muscle-tendon meridians in the body. These exist along the surfaces of the muscles and tendons, running from joint to joint. Unlike the other meridians, these do not connect with any internal organs. They seem to be primarily involved in the gross utilization of energy with which the musculature is associated. Here, however, there is far greater efficiency (that is, minimized effort with increased energy output) than is ordinarily presumed to be normal.

Muscle-tendon meridians originate in the extremities, meet at major joints and end at points ranging throughout the torso and head. Knowing the tendon routes well and energizing them will greatly increase the muscle-tendon-fascia tone and improve the range of movement, or radius.

1. The Lung Muscle-Tendon Meridian (Figure 5—4)

This meridian has its origin at the end of the thumb. Looking at a person standing and facing you with his arms at the sides of his body and the palms facing forward, the meridian would be seen as a line

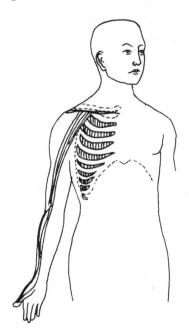

FIGURE 5-4

The Lung Muscle-Tendon Meridian

that extends up along the outer side of the bones of the thumb to the outer side of the wrist. It then ascends up the outerside of the forearm to the crook of the arm and, rising up the biceps, crosses over to and enters the chest, coming out again at the sterno-clavicular joint. From there, it extends across the collar bone to the front deltoid, while another branch extends downward into the chest, sending still other branches down to the diaphragm.

2. The Large Intestine Muscle-Tendon Meridian (Figure 5-5)

Again, picture a person who is standing and facing you. Now his arms are at his sides with the palms facing inward to the torso. Beginning at the end of the index finger, this meridian travels up along what is then the outerside of the forearm to the outer portion of the crook in the arm. There it continues to ascend along the outer side of the upper arm to the side deltoid and then splits into two branches. One goes back over the trapezius muscle, descending down between the spinal column and scapula and extending up along the backbone to about midway of the length of the neck. The other travels across the lower surface of the trapezius and then to the sternocleidomas-

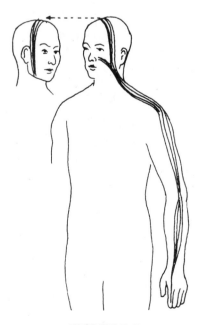

FIGURE 5-5

The Large Intestine Muscle-Tendon Meridian

toid muscle on its way to the face, where it splits again at the jaw line. One short branch runs to the corner of the nose, the other travels up along the side of the face, passing through the side of the forehead on its way over the top of the head and down a similar route to the opposite jaw, where it finally anchors.

3. The Stomach Muscle-Tendon Meridian (Figure 5–6)

This meridian is somewhat more elaborate, starting at the third toe and sometimes the second and fourth, too. The meridian runs up the lower surface of the foot to about the level of the ankle. From there it splits into two branches. One goes up the middle of the lower leg to the outside of the knee. The other, running laterally to the first, continues to the hip joint and then up over the ilial crest (upper part of the pelvis) to continue on around to the back where it crosses the lower ribs and joins with an extension of the meridian that runs along

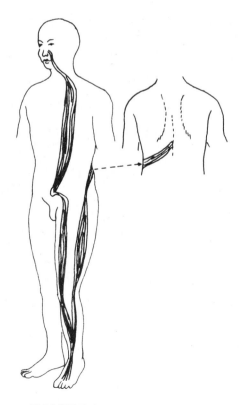

FIGURE 5-6

The Stomach Muscle-Tendon Meridian   267

the backbone from the sacrum to about the level of the collar bone. Returning to the more medially located branch, we see that it continues up to the top of the thigh and veers in towards the pubic bone. There it enters the abdomen and emerges again above the cavity of the collar bone. Next, it travels up the side of the neck and jaw, where it splits in two. One branch veers forward towards the corner of the mouth, ascending up along the side of the nose to the corner of the eye. The other goes up along the jaw line to a point in front of the ear at the temple.

4. The Spleen Muscle-Tendon Meridian (Figure 5–7)

With the figure standing and facing you, this meridian is seen as originating at the middle and end of the big toe. It then runs along the middle of the foot and ascends to the internal malleolus (hammer-shaped bone on each side of the ankle). From there it continues up-

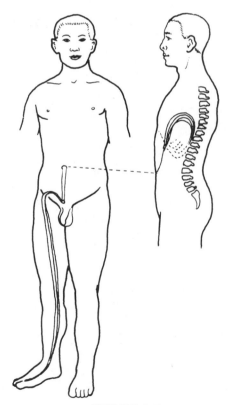

FIGURE 5-7

The Spleen Muscle-Tendon Meridian

ward along the middle of the shin, passing the middle of the knee. Then it travels upward, beginning at the middle of the thigh and sweeping across it to end at a point on the groin. It then turns in toward the pubic bone and rises straight up to the navel. Veering off laterally, it crosses the abdomen, ending at a point just below the nipple, where it then enters into the chest. Another branch runs through a point located at the pubic bone, to the coccygeal region where it ascends the mid-line of the backbone to about the level of the tops of the scapulae.

5. The Heart Muscle-Tendon Meridian (Figure 5–8)

With the person standing with his arms at the sides of his body and the palms facing forward, this meridian begins at the lateral tip of the pinky finger. From there, it ascends to the middle of the wrist, continuing upward along the middle of the forearm to the crook of the arm. Traveling upward and medially, it runs to the armpit and then crosses the pectoral muscle at about the level of the nipple, joins at the mediastinum (the partition between the two pleural sacs of the chest, extending from the sternum to the thoracic vertebrae and downward to the diaphragm) and runs straight down to the navel.

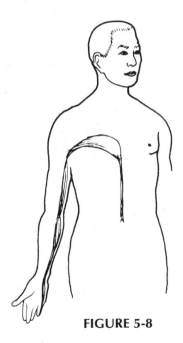

FIGURE 5-8

The Heart Muscle-Tendon Meridian   269

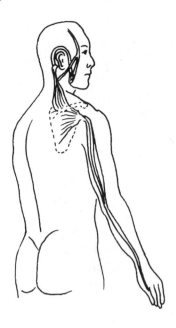

FIGURE 5-9

The Small Intestine Muscle-Tendon Meridian

6. The Small Intestine Muscle-Tendon Meridian (Figure 5–9)

With the person standing and facing away from you with his arms at the sides of his body and the palms facing forward, this meridian begins at the tip of the little finger. Ascending up along the back of that finger to a point on the wrist just above it, it continues up along the middle of the forearm, joining its upper arm extension in the middle of the elbow. Proceeding up the middle of the upper arm, it unites with its neck and ear extension behind the armpit. Ascending and descending, tracing out a pattern like a Z on its side, it continues up and over the trapezius, crossing the neck and connecting at the mastoid process with a small branch entering the ear. Another branch loops up and over the ear and then dips down to end at a point on the jaw below that is slightly behind the level of the outer corner of the eye. It then ascends, passing very close to the outer corner of the eye as it travels to the forehead, uniting with the muscle-tendon meridian extension of the mastoid process at the temple.

Still another branch issues out of the point at the mastoid process, ascending the previously described branch that crosses the forehead on its way to the temple.

7. The Bladder Muscle-Tendon Meridian (Figure 5–10)

Looking at a standing figure faced away from you, the bladder meridian begins in the small toe. Running along the outer side of the foot, it rises and joins with the external malleolus.

It then ascends to and joins the lateral corner of the popliteal fossa (or cavity behind the knee), while a branch extends downward from the external malleolus to join at the heel. Then it runs up along the calf and joins at the back of the knee. From there, it ascends to the middle of the buttocks, while at the same time extending downward along the middle of the calf to the heel. From the buttocks it ascends along the mid-line of the backbone to the nape of the neck, continuing upward to join with the occiput (the lower back part of the skull). It then continues upward across the crown of the head to unite with a point at the side of the nose near the inner corner of the eye. A branch arches along the line of the eyebrow and swoops down to the cheekbone. Then, continuing downward, it extends to the lower jaw, the throat and onto the chest, passing under the armpit to angle up to and join with the line that ascends the back bone. A small branch extends up out of this extension to the backbone, rising at an angle out of the region of the scapula to unite in the shoulder. There is also a branch that extends out of the nape of the neck to unite with the root of the tongue. Finally, a short branch extends from the line coming up and out from under the armpit to join at the mastoid process.

8. The Kidney Muscle-Tendon Meridian (Figure 5–11)

Looking at the back of a standing figure with the left heel lifted, the meridian is seen to start under his little toe. From there it travels along the spleen meridian and curves up at the arch of the foot, passing the underside of the ankle and uniting with the calf extension of

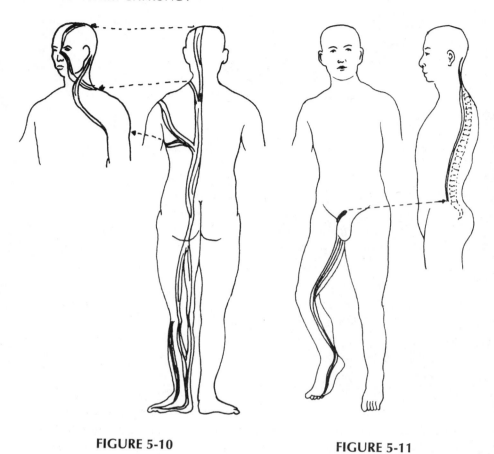

FIGURE 5-10

FIGURE 5-11

The Bladder Muscle-Tendon Meridian

The Kidney Muscle-Tendon Meridian

the muscle-tendon meridian at the Achilles tendon. Continuing to ascend the middle of the calf, it unites again at the middle of the popliteal fossa (cavity behind the knee) joining with the bladder meridian.

Viewing the same standing figure from the front, the kidney meridian is seen to continue up along the inner side of the thigh along with the spleen muscle meridian. It unites at the pubic bone, continuing a short way up to the navel. From the pubic bone it goes through to the coccyx, where it ascends the backbone to connect with the occiput and join with the bladder meridian.

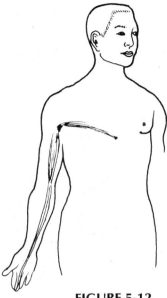

FIGURE 5-12

The Pericardium Muscle-Tendon Meridian

9. The Pericardium Muscle-Tendon Meridian (Figure 5–12)

Facing a standing figure with his arms at his sides and the palms of the hands facing forward, the meridian begins at the middle fingers. It then rises up the mid-line of the forearm and upper arm, passing through the middle of the palm, the crook of the arm, the point of attachment of the front deltoid and then into the armpit. From there it spreads out into the chest both ventrally and dorsally.

10. The Triple Warmer Muscle-Tendon Meridian (Figure 5–13)

Observing a standing figure from the rear with his arms at his sides and the palms of the hands facing forward, the meridian is seen to begin at the end of the fourth finger. It rises to a point directly above it at the wrist and goes up the forearm to the elbow. Then, it travels up the middle of the upper arm, over the trapezius to the neck, where it joins the small intestine meridian. One branch goes to the jaw and connects with the root of the tongue, while the extension of the main

273

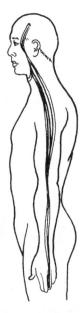

FIGURE 5-13

The Triple Warmer Muscle-Tendon Meridian

meridian rises past the teeth to the ear. There it shifts forward to the outer corner of the eye and continues up past the temple to the upper part of the hairline.

11. The Gall Bladder Muscle-Tendon Meridian (Figure 5–14)

Here, when we view the figure from the side, we find that the meridian begins at the outer side of the end of the fourth toe. From there it angles up along the lower leg, sending out a branch to the outer side of the knee. Continuing up the thigh, it disperses another branch at S–32 and, continuing upward, sends out yet another branch that runs to the anus. It then ascends along the side of the body and rises in front of the shoulder, uniting with the muscle-tendon meridian extension that leads to the breast at the supraclavicular fossa. A slightly divergent point just below this bulges forward, where it links with the breast. The main meridian continues upward, rising up behind the

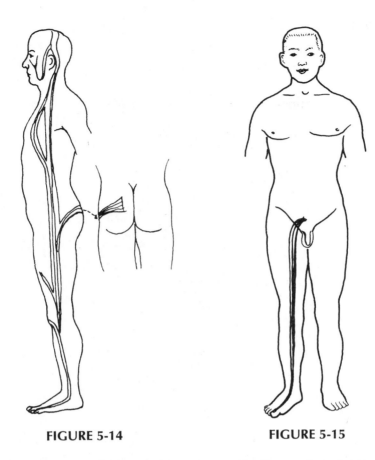

FIGURE 5-14   **FIGURE 5-15**

The Gall Bladder Muscle-Tendon Meridian   **The Liver Muscle-Tendon Meridian**

ear to the crown of the head. It also descends in front of the ear to the side of the jaw from where it ascends again to the corner of the nose, while another branch travels up to the outside corner of the eye.

12. The Liver Muscle-Tendon Meridian (Figure 5–15)

Here we view the standing figure facing us. The meridian starts at the big toe and connects in front of the internal malleolus. It then rises up the lower leg along the tibia (the inner and larger of the two bones of the lower leg) and joins on the inner side of the knee. Finally it sweeps up the thigh and unites at the pubic bone, thereby connecting with all the other muscle meridians.

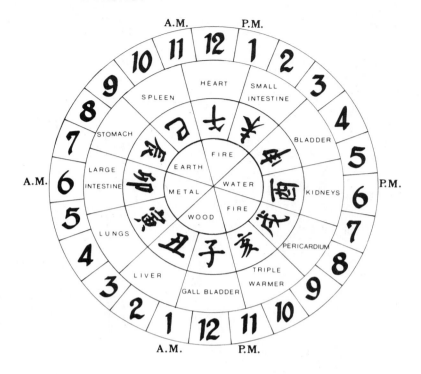

FIGURE 5-16

Timetable of CHI Flow to the Organs

If you want to strengthen a particular muscle-tendon meridian, you can practice by using a CHI timetable. For example, if you want to strengthen the Liver Muscle-Tendon Meridian, it is best to practice at 1:30–3:30 a.m.

6. DEVELOPING A DAILY ROUTINE

If you practice the Six Healing Sounds (as described in *Taoist Ways to Transform Stress into Vitality*) just before going to bed, you will sleep more soundly and awaken earlier and more refreshed. Upon awakening, do not suddenly jump out of bed. Allow your engine (your body) to warm up a little first. Switching into high gear as soon as you get up can be disruptive and damaging to your entire system. If you are in the habit of bouncing out of bed in the morning as soon as you awaken, even though you may experience vitality, lie in bed awhile instead and practice the Inner Smile, allowing the energy to flow into your Microcosmic Orbit, and you will be amazed at how much your health and overall progress will improve. Continue with Chi Self-Massage (as described in *Chi Self-Massage: The Taoist Way of Rejuvenation*). If you are pressed for time, practice Chi Self-Massage while sitting on the toilet seat. It is not necessary to set aside time to do these practices since you can combine them with other activities. After diligently spending time in the Healing Tao System, you will easily be able to realize differences in your general well-being.

You should drink some water when you get up, but not to excess. Drink as much as you feel is comfortable. Imbibing too much water can make you feel nauseated and even damage your kidneys. For drinking purposes it is wise to use a water filter or distill your water. Water and air are your two most important ingredients to good health and steady progress in this system. If you are worried about losing trace minerals through distillation, use tap water to cook with. Then you will have your minerals, too. Make sure that the tap water is filtered, at least through a simple mesh. Make sure that the air that you breathe is filtered as well whenever possible. The "Bionaire" air filter is a good choice because, in addition to filtering the air, it has an ion emitter.

Practice the Iron Shirt exercises you have learned in this book, and in a short time you will find that it all fits together quite easily and becomes as ordinary, and yet as necessary, as brushing your teeth. You will, in other words, begin another good habit. To develop the daily practice of Iron Shirt, it will serve you well to realize that you do not need to do all of the exercises or breath alignment every day. On those days that you practice, it is best to do so early in the morning when you arise. Design a schedule that works for you. You might be able to devote no more than five or ten minutes to an activity, but do it. Rising twenty minutes or a half hour earlier in the morning will improve your whole life. In fact, in a short time you will discover that you need less sleep and have more strength and energy. At the same time, you will find that your activities, both before and after practice, will become more efficient and, therefore, you will derive more benefit, even though you spend what might seem like only a little time in actual practice.

You can create, individually, a schedule to fit your time allowance. A recommended schedule to follow might be:

MONDAY: Embracing the Tree for approximately six to seven minutes, followed by Holding the Golden Urn and the Horse Stance Using a Wall.

TUESDAY: Embracing the Tree, the Turtle and Buffalo and the Horse Stance Using a Wall.

WEDNESDAY: Embracing the Tree, the Turtle and Buffalo, plus the Phoenix and Door Hanging.

THURSDAY: Embracing the Tree, the Phoenix, the Iron Bridge, and the Backbend.

FRIDAY: Embracing the Tree, the Iron Bridge, the Iron Bar and the Warrior Poses.

SATURDAY and SUNDAY: Embracing the Tree, or rest for both days before beginning the cycle again. You may also decide to start the schedule over on Saturday. It is important to remember to start gradually, practicing only fifteen or twenty minutes to a half hour per day.

Iron Shirt can be practiced at any time. Once you master using the mind to bring CHI to the various parts of the organs, you will find it very useful and you will be able to use the CHI energy anytime that you want or need it.

If, for example, you are riding in a car, on a train, or in a plane and you feel back pain, you can bring the energy to the back by pulling up the anus and bringing the energy to the kidneys, or simply by contracting the back muscles. Squeeze and release, squeeze and release and you will find that the pain or stiffness will go away. You will feel energized immediately. In this way you can help the organs that need to be exercised.

Squeeze in some practice whenever you find some time during the day. It does not have to be any particular time and/or place. When you are standing on line, for example, with time on your hands, you can practice the elongation of the spine by pressing the legs down with the sensation of screwing them into the ground. Pull your head up at the same time and push the spine down. Once you master the practice, you can use it in any way that you want.

Do not practice too close to bedtime or you will not be able to sleep. If you feel any discomfort during your practice, consult any Taoist Certified Instructor. If the problem still exists, consult a qualified physician. Remember that exercise is a tool. To misuse such a tool can be harmful. Iron Shirt Chi Kung is not meant to be harmful and will not be if used in the proper way. The exercises have been clearly outlined, as well as the side effects and how to prevent them. If the instructions are followed properly, there will be no problems. People have been practicing this system for many thousands of years successfully.

7. THE IRON SHIRT CHI KUNG EXPERIENCE

A. Testimonials from Advanced Iron Shirt Students

Gunther Weil, Doctor of Psychology

I have been a student of spiritual practice for many years. I was involved for a very long time with the Gurdjieff work as a practitioner. In 1978 my teacher died and I decided to step out of that teaching which, by then, I'd been involved in for some fourteen years. I began studying Taoist work, particularly Tai Chi and then Chi Kung, studying the latter with Don Ahn. In September of 1980, I met Master Chia and learned to practice the Microcosmic Orbit, Seminal Kung Fu, Tai Chi Chi Kung and now, Iron Shirt. The approach taken in teaching Iron Shirt is extremely precise and has provided what was lacking in my previous experience of Chi Kung. Although my health had improved enormously in my earlier experiences, and I had a great deal of energy, I had reached the point of feeling stuck and blocked. I hadn't made any progress in a year. I feel that the Iron Shirt teaching has been very helpful in getting me going again.

Roberta Prada, Opera Singer

As a classically trained singer, I find the Iron Shirt practices, in combination with the Microcosmic Orbit meditation and the Six Healing Sounds, to be of great benefit to my technique. Specifically, my goals for my singing include a free and easy vocal mechanism and an ability to feel grounded and centered while performing. Since beginning the Taoist practices, I have achieved the relaxation of my jaw, the lowering of my breathing, and the ability to search out areas of tension in my body, so that I can release them and allow the free flow of energy throughout my body. The more tissues resonate freely along the paths of vocal production, the more beautiful and powerful the sound becomes, and the production of that sound becomes more precise and effortless. This is true for me. It would be difficult to attribute these results to Iron Shirt alone, since I continually study with a voice teacher as well, and perform regularly. However, I am certain that the degree of body alignment, delicate coordination, physical and mental power, and the ability to still myself, have enhanced my ability to achieve the goals I have set for myself in my art with greater naturalness, precision, clarity and beauty of sound. Ideally, I would like to see courses in these arts form part of the studies offered in conservatories and professional schools as part of the body movement/ breathing curriculum. Tai Chi is already taught in these settings in England. Once the exercises are learned, they can be used in free moments anywhere: on tour, in a dressing room, in small spaces, without equipment, and without a teacher. They are practical and of lasting value.

I would heartily recommend the Microcosmic Orbit meditation, Iron Shirt and Tai Chi to singers, actors, conductors, instrumentalists and dancers as a valuable adjunct to professional studies.

B. Interview of Iron Shirt Practitioner Michael Winn, conducted by John Zielinsky, Instructor

John: Can you tell me when you first started Iron Shirt?

Michael: I first studied Iron Shirt a little over two years ago. Before that, I was doing Kundalini Yoga which involves a lot of breathing and intense energy. I found Iron Shirt to be even more intense because the air was packed inside, held and circulated internally, whereas with the other practices, I breathed in and out and slowly moved the energy around using various sounds. In the beginning I found that I had too much energy in my head for doing Iron Shirt, partly as a result of my other practices. When I started to do Iron Shirt, my face would get very red. As I got better at it, doing it every day, I started to get the energy more rooted, or grounded. I discovered that when a practice is done properly, you are mixing energy from the air with what is in the body, holding it inside where it is somewhat warm, and mixing this with the energy from the ground which is cool. It took me a while to really get the energy down out of my head, and relax before I could begin to practice and feel like I was drawing in some full energy, mixing it and circulating it around.

John: How long after practicing Iron Shirt I did you begin practicing Iron Shirt II and Iron Shirt III? Also, how long do you practice? How frequently every day during all that time, and how much do you now practice?

Michael: I practice every day, almost without fail. I studied the Iron Shirt II a few months later, and Iron Shirt III a year or so after that. I continued doing the Iron Shirt I, even when I did the Iron Shirt II or III. I did not continue with the Iron Shirt II practice because I found that the Iron Shirt I and the Iron Shirt III were sufficient. Iron Shirt III, of course, added another level to my practice. A lot of people do not practice Iron Shirt I long enough to get to the other levels. In fact, what I found out in going through the stages of Iron Shirt I is that it is related to all of the other meditation practices, but as your energy gets more refined and you start to pack the energy in your body more, you feel a different quality to the energy as it circulates around. When I really had it right, I could feel a kind of cool radiant heat emanating out of my body. It was not an electric energy. It was mixed with the Yin energy and properly refined. It left my body feeling that it was together, really flowing, giving me a nice energy throughout the day.

The other sensation started happening after a year and a half as I was beginning to take longer, before doing Iron Shirt I, before packing, to stand and relax more down to the earth. This allowed me to take more cool energy in. I would begin spontaneously to do the full Microcosmic Orbit, down to the leg roots into the ground, bringing the energy back up the front of my legs to the perineum, back to the spine, around the top of my head and rooting to the ground again. As I looked back into the ground, I would then do the Microcosmic Orbit a full body length into the ground below me. In other words, I was pretending that I was buried underground and my head was right at the surface of the earth. I would circulate the energy through myself standing under the ground. I found a very rooted, cool energy and could visualize myself and my energy in the ground below. I pulled the energy back into my body before I even began to pack. I found myself already getting rooted, just with my mind.

Also, at one point, spontaneously, I started seeing a variety of crystals at various points within my body, and in the body in the ground that I was circulating the energy through. This would add another quality to Iron Shirt: refining energy. My practice then continued at a much higher level of energy.

What I finally realized is that when you do the Iron Shirt and you are circulating the energy around in the Microcosmic Orbit, you are also pulling in the earth energy and circulating it around in your body before sending it back down. This is what rooting is about.

John: The variation underground, was that yours or from Master Chia?

Michael: Actually, I asked him about it and he said you could do that when you work from a very high level, and even visualize yourself five body lengths down. I started off visualizing myself all the way down to the center of the earth and pulling earth energy out from there. Then I asked him about it. He said try something closer in the beginning. I found that this position at the center of the earth also worked, but Master Chia warned me that the center of the earth is very molten and I might pull out some very hot energy. It has the same effect though.

I have really begun to notice in whatever I do that there is CHI in my bones. When I am doing Tai Chi, I begin to feel my skeleton with a dense, glowing energy in it. This is what lets me know that the energy is not just in my body anymore, or just in my head. When you swing your arm, the feeling is that the flesh and the blood are really light and not quite there, but in the center you can feel steel, an energy that is packed in. I think you get the same sensation from Tai Chi or anything else, but doing the Iron Shirt III speeds the process up a hundred times faster. I think the main things to caution against are not to get too much hot energy into your head or into your heart. When you hold the energy in for a long time and circulate it around, it can strain your heart. The important thing, then, is to start gradually and bring your body up so that it can handle the energy until you can move it around comfortably.

John: Do you relax after you exercise and walk?

Michael: Yes. This is very important. Some days Iron Shirt I is so intense that I do not do anything else. The energy that I have pulled in and circulated through my body is enough for me to digest and work with. I do not do any other practice, not Tai Chi, not anything, because my body has been fed, even stuffed. In fact, I have to sit down and digest the meal.

John: Have you noticed any specific health benefits related to the Iron Shirt practice?

Michael: Yes. In my other practice with Kundalini Yoga, the energy would be very high, but it would leak out of my body. I noticed in the winter that I would be cold. I was becoming very Yin. It was a very Yang practice, but it used up the energy in my body. I notice now with Iron Shirt that my body is much warmer in the winter. I can withstand the weather, the elements. I was already becoming very healthy as far as not getting very much illness or sickness from Kundalini Yoga, but I feel that this has further increased my abilities to fight off flus or colds, or any similar illness. At one time, four or five family members were visiting me and they all came down with the flu and were out for a week. I felt it try to come into my body for a day or so, and I felt very weak. I was able to push it out. I think that packing the CHI inside your body leaves no room for the bacteria, viruses, etc., once the CHI has been built up to a certain level.

John: One other question about your practices: When you practiced Iron Shirt, did you have someone do the pushing to develop the rooting?

Michael: I was living alone and often did not have anyone with me, which is unfortunate. Periodically I would go over to the center and get pushed again and found that I was breaking at the waist, for example, because I did not have my posture quite right. There are small corrections you really need to make. They probably slowed down my progress in getting it right. I was still studying the energy and still packing it in, but there is no benefit to doing so if you do not do it perfectly. So I would say that it is good to get pushed.

John: Michael, I know you lead a busy life and you have a lot of mental activity; do you find that Iron Shirt III helps you to cope with stress from day to day life? Does it help you on a mental level as well as a physical?

Michael: Yes. Sometimes when I am writing, I will work for fifteen or sixteen hours a day. When I feel that I have used up my CHI, my energy, and my brain is not functioning enough, I will do some Iron

Shirt to get the energy going again. At times, I do not want to sleep, I want to keep going and keep pushing myself, but I do not think this is the right way to live. It is smarter to live simply. However, sometimes you find yourself in the situation of a deadline and, yes, it definitely helps to relieve the stress.

John: Do you have any other general comments about your Iron Shirt practice?

Michael: I have seen other kinds of Chi Kung, and they involve movement and inhaling and exhaling with those movements, and I think those other Chi Kung are valid and powerful. However, I think that ultimately, this is a higher Chi Kung because it is more internal. In other words, it does not rely on continual breathing, or continued movement of any sort. You do breathe in in the beginning, but as you move along to higher levels of the Iron Shirt Chi Kung, you do not even have to bring in your breath, but can just draw in the energy with your mind, pack it and circulate it around. Movement with your mind emphasizes the internal aspects of the energy; it is also more integrating. That can be a problem in the beginning for a novice whose mind is not integrating with his CHI, and he cannot move his CHI around with his mind. He needs to use more breathing and more movement. I think that if a person sticks with it, it will come in time.

C. Personal Experiences of Students

• No matter what sort of physical activity I indulge in since I've begun studying here, I feel heat in my arms, legs and back. I'm sure that something has opened up for me.

• I cook for a living and I get cut and nicked a lot at work. I've noticed since coming here that I heal a lot quicker. There's something else. I feel I can store a lot of energy in my back now.

• Iron Shirt makes me feel as though I've discovered myself. I've meditated and used energy in other systems, but they've been nothing like what I've experienced here.

• What I enjoyed the most was the harmony that I found among Iron Shirt Chi Kung that "builds the fire", the meditations to open the channels to enable the "fire" to be transported more fully through the body, and Tai Chi as the means to send the CHI through the channels. It all came together very clearly for me here. My concern has been to preserve the "life-force" in the face of the many influences that attack it in daily life, and how to develop a means of harmonizing and choosing the most life-giving elements that are available. This information has laid out a method that I can easily follow to attain this goal.

• I found Iron Shirt II to be most gratifying. After finishing an Iron Shirt II class, I'd experience a "click" in my hips. This had never happened before. As the week progressed the "clicks" came on sooner and stayed longer. Then, suddenly, three days ago, I discovered that I had new hips and there was an incredible feeling of space throughout my lower abdomen. When I practiced Tai Chi I felt a definite connection between my feet and hips and scapulae. This was something I had heard about and could not enjoy first hand. Now I feel connected all over.

• I first learned about Chi Kung when I was a small boy, reading Kung Fu stories, and I continued to think that it was just story stuff until I came here and found that it is true. Along about April, after practicing Chi Kung for just a couple of months, I had to go to the hospital with a terrible pain at the back near the kidney. At the hospital I was given a morphine shot and I found that my experience with that shot was very similar to the experience I had forcing CHI into my head. So I tried using Iron Shirt to suppress the pain. I didn't have any luck at first, but after a couple of days I was actually able to create the pain-suppressing effects of morphine.

• I have practiced Yoga, Judo and Tai Chi extensively. When I came across Master Chia's book, I sensed that it was just what I'd wanted. I'd had terrible migraines for years. I'm all right now. Before that all the energy had been stuck in my head. I could feel it there, and I could feel it come down when I completed the Orbit. In fact all I had to do to complete the Orbit was bring it down, because I'd actually spent years in my other practices bringing energy up to my head. Now, after three months of practicing Master Chia's Taoist system, I have enormous energy.

• At first Iron Shirt seemed to be too different from the gentleness of the Tai Chi I'd learned. But I learned to recognize the need for the balance that it produces. I feel that I've been learning to use my body, and I see how it is now very different. Soon I will be able to do these exercises on my own, anywhere I need to.

• I feel that I have much more energy now. I can hold my breath twice as long as when I first began to practice. I definitely feel more rooted. I feel energy racing through me.

• I could really feel energy coming up out of the ground doing the Iron Shirt exercises, and I know what it is to be rooted now. Sometimes my legs shake when the energy comes up through them. There's something else, too. My back seems more like one unit. I can inhale more air, and I feel stronger all over.

• I've been practicing meditation for about ten years, primarily a type of Kundalini Yoga meditation practice. It did stress circulation of the energy, but it was only up and down the spine rather than using the front channel. I came across Master Chia's book about six weeks ago and started to practice according to what I read there. I happened to go on a meditation retreat for a month where I was able to practice quite a bit and experience an opening of the Microcosmic Orbit, a deepening of my meditation and a release of blockages that I had been aware of for a number of years. My experience with the Chi Kung thus far has been of an increase in energy flow and a further unblocking of the leg channels.

• I've been studying meditation and martial arts for about nine years and I've always had a complete separation between the two: one being physical and one being spiritual. When I came here, the two were linked together. I'd read about it but had never experienced it, that is, until now. When I lived in San Francisco I thought I had Chi Kung down pat by doing tension exercises, but now as I practice Iron Shirt, I realize that I was going down the wrong road. I was trying to use the mind and to strengthen the muscles, instead of working from the inside structure out.

• For the past 25 years or so I've been involved in martial arts: Karate, Kung Fu and Tai Chi. Through these practices I had experienced various energy centers. I had not been aware of a circuit that had to be completed until I saw it depicted on the cover of Master Chia's book, *Awaken Healing Energy Through the Tao.* I was especially drawn to it because I saw that along that route were some of the centers I had already experienced. When I read the book, I discovered that it answered questions for me that I'd not yet been able to put into words. I began to realize that I must learn to turn my senses inward and to reflect. I recognized that introspection is something we are not ordinarily taught. As I read, I came to believe that this might be what I had been looking for: a method to follow that would allow me to know more about myself.

• I approached the Microcosmic Orbit and Iron Shirt because I was searching for something to cure a serious problem that was unsuccessfully treated previously. I had a four-by-six centimeter duodenal penetrating ulcer. (It's been documented.) And for those who don't know about such things, that's a big ulcer. I also had two crushed discs commonly called kissing vertebrae, from two separate accidents. In addition, I had a genetic curvature of the upper portion of my spine for which I'd had chiropractic adjustments over a period of two years. When I came to inquire about your courses, my digestive system had wound down to a standstill, I had lost about thirty pounds, and my gastroenterologist had told me that I must undergo surgery. In less than four months of practicing Iron Shirt, I actually have scar tissue where the ulcer had existed. I no longer have to take medication, and now I have no back pain, after having experienced it constantly for three years prior to starting this practice. During this period I did nothing but what I've learned here: Iron Shirt each morning, and the Microcosmic Orbit during the day. I have gained twenty-five pounds, and I really do feel that Iron Shirt supplied the real healing power.

• I was introduced to Master Chia through a friend who said that he knew that Master Chia could help me get rid of bad headaches. I had seen Chinese, French and American doctors and none of them could do anything to help me with a problem that had made me miserable for almost fifteen years. After three days with Master Chia, I completed the Orbit and gradually I found my headaches were subsiding.

• I studied some Tai Kwan Do and I'm presently studying Praying Mantis Kung Fu. I became interested in the internal Kung Fu through a friend of mine. As soon as he told me about it, I was interested. I went to learn Tai Chi at the time and learned very fierce breathing exercises. It did seem to get energy going but after practicing it I didn't feel as energetic as I do here. The surprising thing about Master Chia's system is that it's so simple to do, and yet, it's so effective in doing what it's supposed to do. I feel it inside my navel as opposed to feeling it in my stomach or my elbow or different parts of my body. I also find that it helps my martial art practice.

• I have been practicing some martial arts from time to time, especially Hsing Yi, and have sought out internal practices. Your system is by far the best that I have found and I want to thank you for it. In fact, it intergrates Kundalini Yoga and some Western practices, integrating the uses of the centers and the meridians. It is excellent and I want to continue with it.

• I've practiced martial arts, meditation and a number of spiritual disciplines for around eight or nine years and, last spring, I took Master Chia's Microcosmic Orbit workshop. I had the personal experience of feeling the CHI travel through the basic meridians and a number of acupuncture points. I was surprised because before, they were just points in books to me. I thought maybe you could influence that energy with needles, but I never believed you could feel it. I look forward to practicing more and more Iron Shirt and deepening the sensation of the energy and the experience.

• Before coming here I had experienced energy in my body, but I didn't know what to do with it; it seemed very scattered. Through the structure that Master Chia offers, I now have a means of control that I never had before. My background is in martial arts and in meditation for about the past five years. Iron Shirt is something I've never seen offered anywhere else, and I feel it's invaluable to anyone who is doing any martial arts, especially a dynamic type, which can easily throw your body out of alignment or else lead to damaged organs. It's become apparent that if I know how to use this type of energy that I get in Iron Shirt, I feel my risks of sustaining damages are greatly lessened.

• I still have a long way to go to develop any rooting power, but I do feel stronger, especially in my back.

• You brought up something a little while ago about people having more difficulty in dealing with pleasure than with pain. Well, I'd been meditating twice a day during my vacation and got so high that I just couldn't stand it. My whole body was like golden light. I had to back away from the practice. I just wasn't ready for it. This stuff is really authentic. I am very convinced. There's another thing I'd like to say about this practice. I am an acupuncturist and have no trouble getting patients these days. I never even have to think about soliciting clients. They just show up. My work is more effective, efficient and clear.

• I find myself growing, now that I have discovered this teaching, and I've discovered my body. I've already helped my body immensely. I want to learn everything that I can that relates to these methods, now. The effects are too convincing. It's like coming across the answers to everything.

• I came from another system that I felt was very good, in fact, perfect. So I really wasn't looking for anything else, except that I was curious to know about this other system. I found the Healing Tao exciting and very different. As I went into it and felt so much energy running around in my channels, I began to miss some of those simpler powerful ethics of my earlier meditations. It took me a while of practicing the Taoist meditations on a daily basis to understand that in the Taoist approach, I was making use of sources of energy that I had, in my earlier system, not tapped. While previously I had been achieving one sort of intensity of energy, I find that through Tai Chi and Iron Shirt, I can hold that energy in my body rather that just having a temporary experience that might come on from a lot of chanting or breathing exercises.

THE INTERNATIONAL HEALING TAO SYSTEM

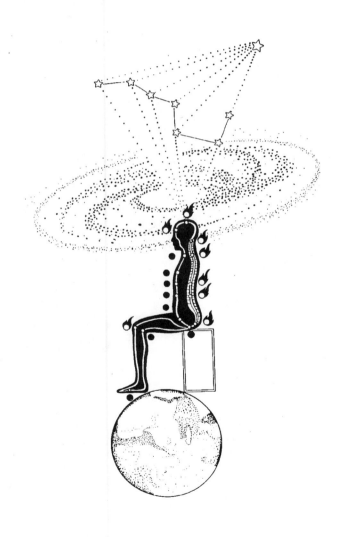

The Goal of the Taoist Practice

The Healing Tao is a practical system of self-development that enables the individual to complete the harmonious evolution of the physical, mental, and spiritual planes the achievement of spiritual independence.

Through a series of ancient Chinese meditative and internal energy exercises, the practitioner learns to increase physical energy, release tension, improve health, practice self-defense, and gain the ability to heal oneself and others. In the process of creating a solid foundation of health and well-being in the physical body, the basis for developing one's spiritual independence is also created. While learning to tap the natural energies of the Sun, Moon, Earth, and Stars, a level of awareness is attained in which a solid spiritual body is developed and nurtured.

The ultimate goal of the Tao practice is the transcendence of physical boundaries through the development of the soul and the spirit within man.

International Healing Tao Course Offerings

There are now many International Healing Tao centers in the United States, Canada, Bermuda, Germany, Netherlands, Switzerland, Austria, France, Spain, India, Japan, and Australia offering personal instruction in various practices including the Microcosmic Orbit, the Healing Love Meditation, Tai Chi Chi Kung, Iron Shirt Chi Kung, and the Fusion Meditations.

Healing Tao Warm Current Meditation, as these practices are also known, awakens, circulates, directs, and preserves the generative life-force called Chi through the major acupuncture meridians of the body. Dedicated practice of this ancient, esoteric system eliminates stress and nervous tension, massages the internal organs, and restores health to damaged tissues.

Outline of the Complete System of The Healing Tao

Courses are taught at our various centers. Direct all written inquiries to one central address or call:

The Healing Tao Center
P.O. Box 1194
Huntington, NY 11743
516-367-2701

INTRODUCTORY LEVEL I: Awaken Your Healing Light

Course 1: (1) Opening of the Microcosmic Channel; (2) The Inner Smile; (3) The Six Healing Sounds; and (4) Tao Rejuvenation—Chi Self-Massage.

INTRODUCTORY LEVEL II: Development of Internal Power

Course 2: Healing Love: Seminal and Ovarian Kung Fu.

Course 3: Iron Shirt Chi Kung; Organs Exercise and Preliminary Rooting Principle. The Iron Shirt practice is divided into three workshops: Iron Shirt I, II, and III.

Course 4: Fusion of the Five Elements, Cleansing and Purifying the Organs, and Opening of the Six Special Channels. The Fusion practice is divided into three workshops: Fusion I, II, and III.

Course 5: Tai Chi Chi Kung; the Foundation of Tai Chi Chuan. The Tai Chi practice is divided into seven workshops: (1) Original Thirteen Movements' Form (five directions, eight movements); (2) Fast Form of Discharging Energy; (3) Long Form (108 movements); (4) Tai Chi Sword; (5) Tai Chi Knife; (6) Tai Chi Short and Long Stick; (7) Self-Defense Applications and Mat Work.

Course 6: Taoist Five Element Nutrition; Taoist Healing Diet.

INTRODUCTORY LEVEL III: The Way of Radiant Health

Course 7: Healing Hands Kung Fu; Awaken the Healing Hand—Five Finger Kung Fu.

Course 8: Chi Nei Tsang; Organ Chi Transformation Massage. This practice is divided into three levels: Chi Nei Tsang I, II, and III.

Course 9: Space Dynamics; The Taoist Art of Energy Placement.

INTERMEDIATE LEVEL: Foundations of Spiritual Practice

Course 10: Lesser Enlightenment Kan and Li: Opening of the Twelve Channels; Raising the Soul, and Developing the Energy Body.

Course 11: Greater Enlightenment Kan and Li: Raising the Spirit and Developing the Spiritual Body.

Course 12: Greatest Enlightenment: Educating the Spirit and the Soul; Space Travel.

ADVANCED LEVEL: The Immortal Tao (The Realm of Soul and Spirit)

Course 13: Sealing of the Five Senses.

Course 14: Congress of Heaven and Earth.

Course 15: Reunion of Heaven and Man.

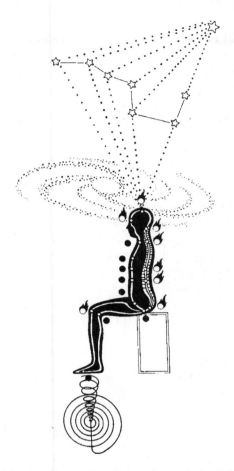

Course Descriptions of The Healing Tao System

INTRODUCTORY LEVEL I: Awaken Your Healing Light

Course 1:

A. The first level of the Healing Tao system involves opening the Microcosmic Orbit within yourself. An open Microcosmic Orbit enables you to expand outward to connect with the Universal, Cosmic Particle, and Earth Forces. Their combined forces are considered by Taoists as the Light of Warm Current Meditation.

Through unique relaxation and concentration techniques, this practice awakens, circulates, directs, and preserves the generative life-force, or Chi, through the first two major acupuncture channels (or meridians) of the body: the Functional Channel which runs down the chest, and the Governor Channel which ascends the middle of the back.

Dedicated practice of this ancient, esoteric method eliminates stress and nervous tension, massages the internal organs, restores health to damaged tissues, increases the consciousness of being alive, and establishes a sense of well-being. Master Chia and certified instructors will assist students in opening the Microcosmic Orbit by passing energy through their hands or eyes into the students' energy channels.

B. *The Inner Smile* is a powerful relaxation technique that utilizes the expanding energy of happiness as a language with which to communicate with the internal organs of the body. By learning to smile inwardly to the organs and glands, the whole body will feel loved and appreciated. Stress and tension will be counteracted, and the flow of Chi increased. One feels the energy descend down the entire length of the body like a waterfall. The Inner Smile will help the student to counteract stress, and help to direct and increase the flow of Chi.

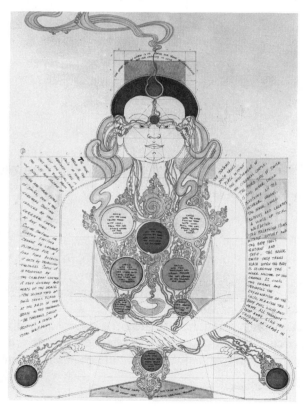

C. *The Six Healing Sounds* is a basic relaxation technique utilizing simple arm movements and special sounds to produce a cooling effect upon the internal organs. These special sounds vibrate specific organs, while the arm movements, combined with posture, guide heat and pressure out of the body. The results are improved digestion, reduced internal stress, reduced insomnia and headaches, and greater vitality as the Chi flow increases through the different organs.

The Six Healing Sounds method is beneficial to anyone practicing various forms of meditation, martial arts, or sports in which there is a tendency to build up excessive heat in the system.

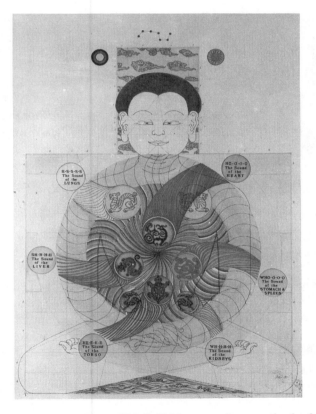

D. *Taoist Rejuvenation—Chi Self-Massage* is a method of hands-on self-healing work using one's internal energy, or Chi, to strengthen and rejuvenate the sense organs (eyes, ears, nose, tongue), teeth, skin, and inner organs. Using internal power (Chi) and gentle external stimulation, this simple, yet highly effective, self-massage technique enables one to dissolve some of the energy blocks and stress points responsible for disease and the aging process. Taoist Rejuvenation dates back 5000 years to the Yellow Emperor's classic text on Taoist internal medicine.

Completion of the Microcosmic Orbit, the Inner Smile, the Six Healing Sounds, and Tao Rejuvenation techniques are prerequisites for any student who intends to study Introductory Level II of the Healing Tao practice.

INTRODUCTORY LEVEL II: Development of Internal Power

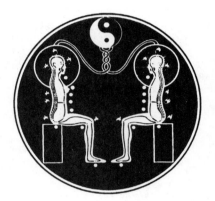

Course 2: *Healing Love: Seminal and Ovarian Kung Fu; Transforming Sexual Energy to Higher Centers, and the Art of Harmonious Relationships*

For more than five thousand years of Chinese history, the "no-outlet method" of retaining the seminal fluid during sexual union has remained a well-guarded secret. At first it was practiced exclusively by the Emperor and his innermost circle. Then, it passed from father to chosen son alone, excluding all female family members. Seminal and Ovarian Kung Fu practices teach men and women how to transform and circulate sexual energy through the Microcosmic Orbit. Rather than eliminating sexual intercourse, ancient Taoist yogis learned how to utilize sexual energy as a means of enhancing their internal practice.

The conservation and transformation of sexual energy during intercourse acts as a revitalizing factor in the physical and spiritual development of both men and women. The turning back and circulating of the generative force from the sexual organs to the higher energy centers of the body invigorates and rejuvenates all the vital functions. Mastering this practice produces a deep sense of respect for all forms of life.

In ordinary sexual union, the partners usually experience a type of orgasm which is limited to the genital area. Through special Taoist techniques, men and women learn to experience a total body orgasm without indiscriminate loss of vital energy. The conservation and transformation of sexual energy is essential for the work required in advanced Taoist practice.

Seminal and Ovarian Kung Fu is one of the five main branches of Taoist Esoteric Yoga.

Course 3: *Iron Shirt Chi Kung; Organs Exercises and Preliminary Rooting Principle*

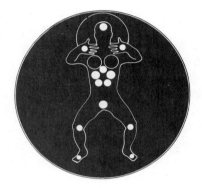

The Iron Shirt practice is divided into three parts: Iron Shirt I, II, and III.

The physical integrity of the body is sustained and protected through the accumulation and circulation of internal power (Chi) in the vital organs. The Chi energy that began to circulate freely through the Microcosmic Orbit and later the Fusion practices can be stored in the fasciae as well as in the vital organs. Fasciae are layers of connective tissues covering, supporting, or connecting the organs and muscles.

The purpose of storing Chi in the organs and muscles is to create a protective layer of interior power that enables the body to withstand unexpected injuries. Iron Shirt training roots the body to the Earth, strengthens the vital organs, changes the tendons, cleanses the bone marrow, and creates a reserve of pure Chi energy.

Iron Shirt Chi Kung is one of the foundations of spiritual practices since it provides a firm rooting for the ascension of the spirit body. The higher the spirit goes, the more solid its rooting to the Earth must be.

Iron Shirt Chi Kung I—Connective Tissues' and Organs' Exercise: On the first level of Iron Shirt, by using certain standing postures, muscle locks, and Iron Shirt Chi Kung breathing techniques, one learns how to draw and circulate energy from the ground. The standing postures teach how to connect the internal structure (bones, muscles, tendons, and fasciae) with the ground so that rooting power is developed. Through breathing techniques, internal power is directed to the organs, the twelve tendon channels, and the fasciae.

Over time, Iron Shirt strengthens the vital organs as well as the tendons, muscles, bones, and marrow. As the internal structure is strengthened through layers of Chi energy, the problems of poor posture and circulation of energy are corrected. The practitioner learns the importance of being physically and psychologically rooted in the Earth, a vital factor in the more advanced stages of Taoist practice.

Iron Shirt Chi Kung II—Tendons' Exercise: In the second level of Iron Shirt, one learns how to combine the mind, heart, bone structure, and Chi flow into one moving unit. The static forms learned in the first level of Iron Shirt evolve at this level into moving postures. The goal of Iron Shirt II is to develop rooting power and the ability to absorb and discharge energy through the tendons. A series of exercises allow the student to change, grow, and strengthen the tendons, to stimulate the vital organs, and to integrate the fasciae, tendons, bones, and muscles into one piece. The student also learns methods for releasing accumulated toxins in the muscles and joints of the body. Once energy flows freely through the organs, accumulated poisons can be discharged out of the body very efficiently without resorting to extreme fasts or special dietary aids.

Iron Shirt Chi Kung I is a prerequisite for this course.

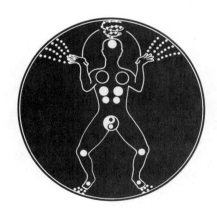

Bone Marrow Nei Kung (Iron Shirt Chi Kung III)—Cleansing the Marrow: In the third level of Iron Shirt, one learns how to cleanse and grow the bone marrow, regenerate sexual hormones and store them in the fasciae, tendons, and marrow, as well as how to direct the internal power to the higher energy centers.

This level of Iron Shirt works directly on the organs, bones, and tendons in order to strengthen the entire system beyond its ordinary capacity. An extremely efficient method of vibrating the internal organs allows the practitioner to shake toxic deposits out of the inner structure of each organ by enhancing Chi circulation. This once highly secret method of advanced Iron Shirt, also known as the Golden Bell System, draws the energy produced in the sexual organs into the higher energy centers to carry out advanced Taoist practices.

Iron Shirt Chi Kung is one of the five essential branches of Taoist Esoteric Practice.

Prior study of Iron Shirt Chi Kung I and Healing Love are prerequisites for this course.

Course 4: *Fusion of the Five Elements,*
Cleansing of the Organs, and
Opening of the Six Special Channels

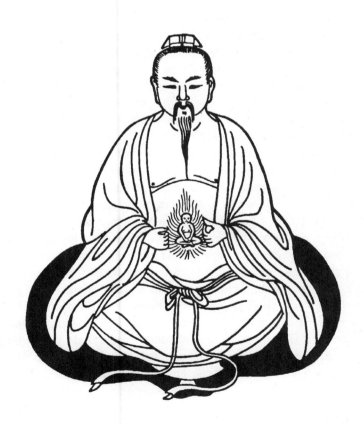

Fusion of the Five Elements and Cleansing of the Organs I, II, and III is the second formula of the Taoist Yoga Meditation of Internal Alchemy. At this level, one learns how the five elements (Earth, Metal, Fire, Wood, and Water), and their corresponding organs (spleen, lungs, heart, liver, and kidneys) interact with one another in three distinct ways: producing, combining, and strengthening. The Fusion practice combines the energies of the five elements and their corresponding emotions into one harmonious whole.

Fusion of the Five Elements I: In this practice of internal alchemy, the student learns to transform the negative emotions of worry, sadness, cruelty, anger, and fear into pure energy. This process is accomplished by identifying the source of the negative emotions within the five organs of the body. After the excessive energy of the emotions is filtered out of the organs, the state of psycho/physical balance is restored to the body. Freed of negative emotions, the pure energy of the five organs is crystallized into a radiant pearl or crystal ball. The pearl is circulated in the body and attracts to it energy from external sources — Universal Energy, Cosmic Particle Energy, and Earth Energy. The pearl plays a central role in the development and nourishment of the soul or energy body. The energy body then is nourished with the pure (virtue) energy of the five organs.

Fusion of the Five Elements II: The second level of Fusion practice teaches additional methods of circulating the pure energy of the five organs once they are freed of negative emotions. When the five organs are cleansed, the positive emotions of kindness, gentleness, respect, fairness, justice, and compassion rise as a natural expression of internal balance. The practitioner is able to monitor his state of balance by observing the quality of emotions arising spontaneously within.

The energy of the positive emotions is used to open the three channels running from the perineum, at the base of the sexual organs, to the top of the head. These channels collectively are known as the Thrusting Channels or Routes. In addition, a series of nine levels called the Belt Channel is opened, encircling the nine major energy centers of the body.

Fusion of Five Elements III: The third level of Fusion practice completes the cleansing of the energy channels in the body by opening the positive and negative leg and arm channels. The opening of the Microcosmic Orbit, the Thrusting Channels, the Belt Channel, the Great Regulator, and Great Bridge Channels makes the body extremely permeable to the circulation of vital energy. The unhindered circulation of energy is the foundation of perfect physical and emotional health.

The Fusion practice is one of the greatest achievements of the ancient

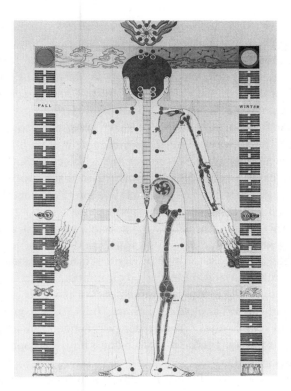

Taoist masters, as it gives the individual a way of freeing the body of negative emotions, and, at the same time, allows the pure virtues to shine forth.

Course 5: *Tai Chi Chi Kung;*
The Foundation
of Tai Chi Chuan

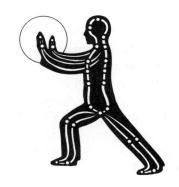

The Tai Chi practice is divided into seven workshops: (1) the Original Thirteen Movements' Form (five directions, eight movements); (2) Fast Form of Discharging Energy; (3) Long Form (108 movements); (4) Tai Chi Sword; (5) Tai Chi Knife; (6) Tai Chi Short and Long Stick; (7) Self-Defense Applications and Mat Work.

Through Tai Chi Chuan the practitioner learns to move the body in one unit, utilizing Chi energy rather than muscle power. Without the circulation of Chi through the channels, muscles, and tendons, the Tai Chi Chuan movements are only physical exercises with little effect on the inner structure of the body. In the practice of Tai Chi Chi Kung, the increased energy flow developed through the Microcosmic Orbit, Fusion work, and Iron Shirt practice is integrated into ordinary movement, so that the body learns more efficient ways of utilizing energy in motion. Improper body movements restrict energy flow causing energy blockages, poor posture, and, in some cases, serious illness. Quite often, back problems are the result of improper posture, accumulated tension, weakened bone structure, and psychological stress.

Through Tai Chi one learns how to use one's own mass as a power to work along with the force of gravity rather than against it. A result of increased body awareness through movement is an increased awareness of one's environment and the potentials it contains. The Tai Chi practitioner may utilize the integrated movements of the body as a means of self-defense in negative situations. Since Tai Chi is a gentle way of exercising and keeping the body fit, it can be practiced well into advanced age because the movements do not strain one's physical capacity as some aerobic exercises do.

Before beginning to study the Tai Chi Chuan form, the student must complete: (1) Opening of the Microcosmic Orbit, (2) Seminal and Ovarian Kung Fu, (3) Iron Shirt Chi Kung I, and (4) Tai Chi Chi Kung.

Tai Chi Chi Kung is divided into seven levels.

Tai Chi Chi Kung I is comprised of four parts:

 a. Mind: (1) How to use one's own mass together with the force of gravity; (2) how to use the bone structure to move the whole body with very little muscular effort; and (3) how to learn and master the thirteen movements so that the mind can concentrate on directing the Chi energy.

 b. Mind and Chi: Use the mind to direct the Chi flow.

 c. Mind, Chi, and Earth force: How to integrate the three forces into one unit moving unimpeded through the bone structure.

 d. Learn applications of Tai Chi for self-defense.

Tai Chi Chi Kung II—Fast Form of Discharging Energy:

 a. Learn how to move fast in the five directions.

 b. Learn how to move the entire body structure as one piece.

 c. Discharge the energy from the Earth through the body structure.

Tai Chi Chi Kung III—Long Form Tai Chi Chuan:

a. Learn the 108 movements form.

b. Learn how to bring Chi into each movement.

c. Learn the second level of self-defense.

d. Grow "Chi eyes."

Tai Chi Chi Kung IV—the Tai Chi Sword.

Tai Chi Chi Kung V—Tai Chi Knife.

Tai Chi Chi Kung VI—Tai Chi Short and Long Stick.

Tai Chi Chi Kung VII—Application of Self-Defense and Mat Work.

Tai Chi Chuan is one of the five essential branches of the Taoist practice.

Course 6: *Taoist Five Element Nutrition; Taoist Healing Diet*

Proper diet in tune with one's body needs, and an awareness of the seasons and the climate we live in are integral parts of the Healing Tao. It is not enough to eat healthy foods free of chemical pollutants to have good health. One has to learn the proper combination of foods according to the five tastes and the five element theory. By knowing one's predominant element, one can learn how to counteract imbalances inherent in one's nature. Also, as the seasons change, dietary needs vary. One must know how to adjust them to fit one's level of activity. Proper diet can become an instrument for maintaining health and cultivating increased levels of awareness.

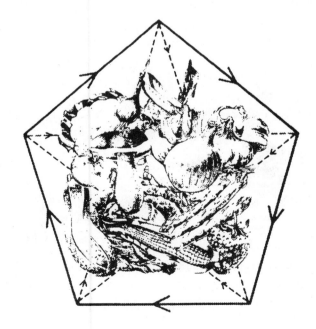

INTRODUCTORY LEVEL III: The Way of Radiant Health

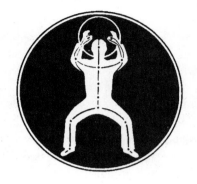

Course 7: *Healing Hands Kung Fu; Awaken the Healing Hand — Five Finger Kung Fu*

The ability to heal oneself and others is one of the five essential branches of the Healing Tao practice. Five Finger Kung Fu integrates both static and dynamic exercise forms in order to cultivate and nourish Chi which accumulates in the organs, penetrates the fasciae, tendons, and muscles, and is finally transferred out through the hands and fingers. Practitioners of body-centered therapies and various healing arts will benefit from this technique. Through the practice of Five Finger Kung Fu, you will learn how to expand your breathing capacity in order to further strengthen your internal organs, tone and stretch the lower back and abdominal muscles, regulate weight, and connect with Father Heaven and Mother Earth healing energy; and you will learn how to develop the ability to concentrate for self-healing.

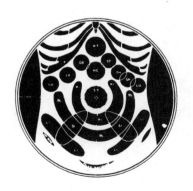

Course 8: *Chi Nei Tsang; Organ Chi Transformation Massage*

The practice is divided into three levels: Chi Nei Tsang I, II, and III.

Chi Nei Tsang, or Organ Chi Transformation Massage, is an entire system of Chinese deep healing that works with the energy flow of the five major systems in the body: the vascular system, the lymphatic system, the nervous system, the tendon/muscle system, and the acupuncture meridian system.

In the Chi Nei Tsang practice, one is able to increase energy flow to specific organs through massaging a series of points in the navel area. In Taoist practice, it is believed that all the Chi energy and the organs, glands, brain, and nervous system are joined in the navel; therefore, energy blockages in the navel area often manifest as symptoms in other parts of the body. The abdominal cavity contains the large intestine, small intestine, liver, gall bladder, stomach, spleen, pancreas, bladder, and sex organs, as well as many lymph nodes. The aorta and vena cava divide into two branches at the navel area, descending into the legs.

Chi Nei Tsang works on the energy blockages in the navel and then follows the energy into the other parts of the body. Chi Nei Tsang is a very deep science of healing brought to the United States by Master Mantak Chia.

Course 9: *Space Dynamics; The Taoist Art of Placement*

Feng Shui has been used by Chinese people and emperors for five thousand years. It combines ancient Chinese Geomancy, Taoist Metaphysics, dynamic Psychology, and modern Geomagnetics to diagnose energy, power, and phenomena in nature, people, and buildings. The student will gain greater awareness of his own present situation, and see more choices for freedom and growth through the interaction of the Five Elements.

INTERMEDIATE LEVEL: Foundations of Spiritual Practice

Course 10: *Lesser Enlightenment (Kan and Li); Opening of the Twelve Channels; Raising the Soul andDeveloping theEnergy Body*

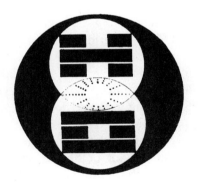

Lesser Enlightenment of Kan and Li (Yin and Yang Mixed): This formula is called *Siaow Kan Li* in Chinese, and involves a literal steaming of the sexual energy (Ching or creative) into life-force energy (Chi) in order to feed the soul or energy body. One might say that the transfer of the sexual energy power throughout the whole body and brain begins with the practice of Kan and Li. The crucial secret of this formula is to reverse the usual sites of Yin and Yang power, thereby provoking liberation of the sexual energy.

This formula includes the cultivation of the root (the Hui-Yin) and the heart center, and the transformation of sexual energy into pure Chi at the navel. This inversion places the heat of the bodily fire beneath the coolness of the bodily water. Unless this inversion takes place, the fire simply moves up and burns the body out. The water (the sexual fluid) has the tendency to flow downward and out. When it dries out, it is the end. This formula reverses normal wasting of energy by the highly advanced method of placing the water in a closed vessel (cauldron) in the body, and then cooking the sperm (sexual energy) with the fire beneath. If the water (sexual energy) is not sealed, it will flow directly into the fire and extinguish it or itself be consumed.

This formula preserves the integrity of both elements, thus allowing the steaming to go on for great periods of time. The essential formula is to never let the fire rise without having water to heat above it, and to never allow the water to spill into the fire. Thus, a warm, moist steam is produced containing tremendous energy and health benefits, to regrow all the glands, the nervous system, and the lymphatic system, and to increase pulsation.

The formula consists of:

1. Mixing the water (Yin) and fire (Yang), or male and female, to give birth to the soul;
2. Transforming the sexual power (creative force) into vital energy (Chi), gathering and purifying the Microcosmic outer alchemical agent;
3. Opening the twelve major channels;
4. Circulating the power in the solar orbit (cosmic orbit);
5. Turning back the flow of generative force to fortify the body and the brain, and restore it to its original condition before puberty;
6. Regrowing the thymus gland and lymphatic system;
7. Sublimation of the body and soul: self-intercourse. Giving birth to the immortal soul (energy body).

Course 11: *Greater Enlightenment (Kan and Li); Raising the Spirit and Developing the Spiritual Body*

This formula comprises the Taoist Dah Kan Li (Ta Kan Li) practice. It uses the same energy relationship of Yin and Yang inversion but

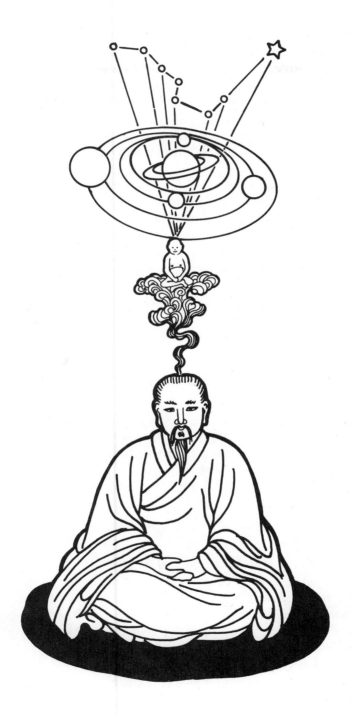

increases to an extraordinary degree the amount of energy that may be drawn up into the body. At this stage, the mixing, transforming, and harmonizing of energy takes place in the solar plexus. The increasing amplitude of power is due to the fact that the formula not only draws Yin and Yang energy from within the body, but also draws the power directly from Heaven and Earth or ground (Yang and Yin, respectively), and adds the elemental powers to those of one's own body. In fact, power can be drawn from any energy source, such as the Moon, wood, Earth, flowers, animals, light, etc.

The formula consists of:

1. Moving the stove and changing the cauldron;
2. Greater water and fire mixture (self-intercourse);
3. Greater transformation of sexual power into the higher level;
4. Gathering the outer and inner alchemical agents to restore the generative force and invigorate the brain;
5. Cultivating the body and soul;
6. Beginning the refining of the sexual power (generative force, vital force, Ching Chi);
7. Absorbing Mother Earth (Yin) power and Father Heaven (Yang) power. Mixing with sperm and ovary power (body), and soul;
8. Raising the soul;
9. Retaining the positive generative force (creative) force, and keeping it from draining away;
10. Gradually doing away with food, and depending on self sufficiency and universal energy;
11. Giving birth to the spirit, transferring good virtues and Chi energy channels into the spiritual body;
12. Practicing to overcome death;
13. Opening the crown;
14. Space travelling.

Course 12: *Greatest Enlightenment (Kan and Li)*

This formula is Yin and Yang power mixed at a higher energy center. It helps to reverse the aging process by re-establishing the thymus glands and increasing natural immunity. This means that healing energy is radiated from a more powerful point in the body, providing greater benefits to the physical and ethereal bodies.

The formula consists of:

1. Moving the stove and changing the cauldron to the higher center;
2. Absorbing the Solar and Lunar power;

3. Greatest mixing, transforming, steaming, and purifying of sexual power (generative force), soul, Mother Earth, Father Heaven, Solar and Lunar power for gathering the Microcosmic inner alchemical agent;
4. Mixing the visual power with the vital power;
5. Mixing (sublimating) the body, soul and spirit.

ADVANCED LEVEL: The Immortal Tao
The Realm of Soul and Spirit
Course 13: *Sealing of the Five Senses*

This very high formula effects a literal transmutation of the warm current or Chi into mental energy or energy of the soul. To do this, we must seal the five senses, for each one is an open gate of energy loss. In other words, power flows out from each of the sense organs unless there is an esoteric sealing of these doors of energy movement. They must release energy only when specifically called upon to convey information.

Abuse of the senses leads to far more energy loss and degradation than people ordinarily realize. Examples of misuse of the senses are as follows: if you look too much, the seminal fluid is harmed; listen too much, and the mind is harmed; speak too much, and the salivary glands are harmed; cry too much, and the blood is harmed; have sexual intercourse too often, and the marrow is harmed, etc.

Each of the elements has a corresponding sense through which its elemental force may be gathered or spent. The eye corresponds to fire; the tongue to water; the left ear to metal; the right ear to wood; the nose to Earth.

The fifth formula consists of:

1. Sealing the five thieves: ears, eyes, nose, tongue, and body;
2. Controlling the heart, and seven emotions (pleasure, anger, sorrow, joy, love, hate, and desire);
3. Uniting and transmuting the inner alchemical agent into life-preserving true vitality;
4. Purifying the spirit;
5. Raising and educating the spirit; stopping the spirit from wandering outside in quest of sense data;
6. Eliminating decayed food, depending on the undecayed food, the universal energy is the True Breatharian.

Course 14: *Congress of Heaven and Earth*

This formula is difficult to describe in words. It involves the incarnation of a male and a female entity within the body of the adept. These two entities have sexual intercourse within the body. It involves the mixing of the Yin and Yang powers on and about the crown of the head, being totally open to receive energy from above, and the regrowth of the pineal gland to its fullest use. When the pineal gland has developed to its fullest potential, it will serve as a compass to tell us in which direction our aspirations can be found. Taoist Esotericism is a method of mastering the spirit, as described in Taoist Yoga. Without the body, the Tao cannot be attained, but with the body, truth can never be realized. The practitioner of Taoism should preserve his physical body with the same care as he would a precious diamond, because it can be used as a medium to achieve immortality. If, however, you do not abandon it when you reach your destination, you will not realize the truth.

This formula consists of:

1. Mingling (uniting) the body, soul, spirit, and the universe (cosmic orbit);
2. Fully developing the positive to eradicate the negative completely;
3. Returning the spirit to nothingness.

Course 15: *Reunion of Heaven and Man*

We compare the body to a ship, and the soul to the engine and propeller of a ship. This ship carries a very precious and very large diamond which it is assigned to transport to a very distant shore. If your ship is damaged (a sick and ill body), no matter how good the engine is, you are not going to get very far and may even sink. Thus, we advise against spiritual training unless all of the channels in the body have been properly opened, and have been made ready to receive the 10,000 or 100,000 volts of super power which will pour down into them. The Taoist approach, which has been passed down to us for over five thousand years, consists of many thousands of methods. The formulae and practices we describe in these books are based on such secret knowledge and the author's own experience during over twenty years of study and of successively teaching thousands of students.

The main goal of Taoists:

1. This level—overcoming reincarnation, and the fear of death through enlightenment;
2. Higher level—the immortal spirit and life after death;
3. Highest level—the immortal spirit in an immortal body. This body functions like a mobile home to the spirit and soul as it moves through the subtle planes, allowing greater power of manifestation.

Healing Tao Books

AWAKEN HEALING ENERGY THROUGH THE TAO

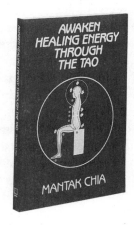

This book reveals for the first time in vivid detail the essentials of the Microcosmic Orbit meditation, a way to awaken your own healing energy. Learn how to strengthen your internal organs and increase circulation through the flow of Chi energy. Included are precise instructions for practice, and detailed illustrations of energy centers, organs, and anatomical structures as well as descriptions of the higher levels of the Taoist meditation system. By Master Mantak Chia. Softbound. 193 pages.

$12.50 plus $1.95 for postage & handling
(Foreign Shipping: Please see page Catalog-39)
Order by Item No. B01

TAOIST SECRETS OF LOVE: CULTIVATING MALE SEXUAL ENERGY

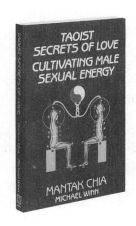

Master Mantak Chia reveals for the first time to the general public the ancient sexual secrets of the Taoist sages. These methods enable men to conserve and transform sexual energy through its circulation in the Microcosmic Orbit, invigorating and rejuvenating the body's vital functions. Hidden for centuries, these esoteric techniques make the process of linking sexual energy and transcendent states of consciousness accessible to the reader.

This revolutionary book teaches:

- Higher Taoist practices for alchemical transmutation of body, mind, and spirit;
- The secret of achieving and maintaining full sexual potency;
- The Taoist "valley orgasm"—pathway to higher bliss;
- How to conserve and store sperm in the body;
- The exchange and balancing of male and female energies within the body, and with one's partner;
- How this can fuel higher achievement in career, personal power, and sports.

This book, co-authored with Michael Winn, is written clearly, and illustrated with many detailed diagrams. Softbound. 250 pages.

$14.95 plus $1.95 for postage & handling
(Foreign Shipping: Please see page Catalog-39)
Order by Item No. B02

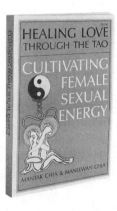

HEALING LOVE THROUGH THE TAO: CULTIVATING FEMALE SEXUAL ENERGY

This book outlines the methods for cultivating female sexual energy. Master Mantak Chia and Maneewan Chia introduce for the first time in the West the different techniques for transforming and circulating female sexual energy. The book teaches:

- The Taoist internal alchemical practices to nourish body, mind, and spirit;
- How to eliminate energy loss through menstruation;
- How to reduce the length of menstruations;
- How to conserve and store ovary energy in the body;
- The exchange and balance of male and female energies within the body, and with one's partner;
- How to rejuvenate the body and mind through vaginal exercises.

Written in clear language by Master Mantak Chia and Maneewan Chia. Published by Healing Tao Books. Softbound. 328 pages.

$14.95 plus $1.95 for postage & handling
(Foreign Shipping: Please see page Catalog-39)
Order by Item No. B06

TAOIST WAYS TO TRANSFORM STRESS INTO VITALITY

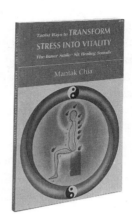

The foundations of success, personal power, health, and peak performance are created by knowing how to transform stress into vitality and power using the techniques of the Inner Smile and Six Healing Sounds, and circulating the smile energy in the Microcosmic Orbit.

The Inner Smile teaches you how to connect with your inner organs, fall in love with them, and smile to them, so that the emotions and stress can be transformed into creativity, learning, healing, and peak performance energy.

The Six Healing Sounds help to cool down the system, eliminate trapped energy, and clean the toxins out of the organs to establish organs that are in peak condition.

By Master Mantak Chia. Published by Healing Tao Books. Softbound. 156 pages.

$10.95 plus $1.95 for postage & handling
(Foreign Shipping: Please see page Catalog-39)
Order by Item No. B03

CHI SELF-MASSAGE: THE TAOIST WAY OF REJUVENATION

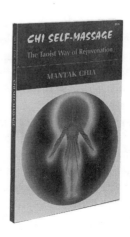

Tao Rejuvenation uses one's internal energy or Chi to strengthen and rejuvenate the sense organs (eyes, ears, nose, tongue), the teeth, the skin, and the inner organs. The techniques are five thousand years old, and, until now, were closely guarded secrets passed on from a Master to a small group of students, with each Master only knowing a small part. For the first time the entire system has been pieced together in a logical sequence, and is presented in such a way that only five or ten minutes of practice daily will improve complexion, vision, hearing, sinuses, gums, teeth, tongue, internal organs, and general stamina. (This form of massage is very different from muscular massage.)

By Master Mantak Chia. Published by Healing Tao Books. Softbound. 176 pages.

$10.95 plus $1.95 for postage & handling
(Foreign Shipping: Please see page Catalog-39)
Order by Item No. B04

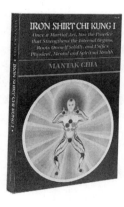

IRON SHIRT CHI KUNG I: INTERNAL ORGANS EXERCISE

The main purpose of Iron Shirt is not for fighting, but to perfect the body, to win great health, to increase performance, to fight disease, to protect the vital organs from injuries, and to lay the groundwork for higher, spiritual work. Iron Shirt I teaches how to increase the performance of the organs during sports, speech, singing, and dancing.

Learn how to increase the Chi pressure throughout the whole system by Iron Shirt Chi Kung breathing, to awaken and circulate internal energy (Chi), to transfer force through the bone structure and down to the ground. Learn how to direct the Earth's power through your bone structure, to direct the internal power to energize and strengthen the organs, and to energize and increase the Chi pressure in the fasciae (connective tissues).

By Master Mantak Chia. Published by Healing Tao Books. Softbound. 320 pages.

$14.95 plus $1.95 for postage & handling
(Foreign Shipping: Please see page Catalog-39)
Order by Item No. B05

BONE MARROW NEI KUNG: IRON SHIRT CHI KUNG III

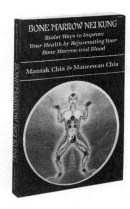

Bone Marrow Nei Kung is a system to cultivate internal power. By absorbing cosmic energy into the bones, the bone marrow is revitalized, blood replenished, and the life-force within is nourished. These methods are known to make the body impervious to illness and disease. In ancient times, the "Steel Body" attained through this practice was a coveted asset in the fields of Chinese medicine and martial arts. Taoist methods of "regrowing" the bone marrow are crucial to rejuvenating the body, which in turn rejuvenates the mind and spirit. This system has not been revealed before, but in this ground-breaking work Master Chia divulges the step-by-step practice of his predecessors.

By Master Mantak Chia and Maneewan Chia. Published by Healing Tao Books. Softbound. 288 pages.

$14.95 plus $1.95 for postage & handling
(Foreign Shipping: Please see page Catalog-39)
Order by Item No. B08

FUSION OF THE FIVE ELEMENTS I

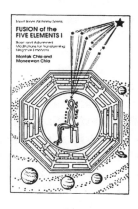

Fusion of the Five Elements I, first in the Taoist Inner Alchemy Series, offers basic and advanced meditations for transforming negative emotions. Based on the Taoist Five Element Theory regarding the five elemental forces of the universe, the student learns how to control negative energies and how to transform them into useful energy. The student also learns how to create a pearl of radiant energy and how to increase its power with additional internal energy (virtue energy) as well as external sources of energy— Universal, Cosmic Particle, and Earth. All combine in a balanced way to prepare the pearl for its use in the creation of an energy body. The creation of the energy body is the next major step in achieving the goal of creating an immortal spirit. Master Mantak Chia leads you, step by step, into becoming an emotionally balanced, controlled, and stronger individual as he offers you the key to a spiritual independence.

$12.95 plus $1.95 for postage & handling
(Foreign Shipping: Please see page Catalog-39)
Order by Item No. B09

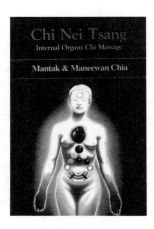

Chi Nei Tsang
(Internal Organ Chi Massage)

Chi Nei Tsang presents a whole new understanding and approach to healing with detailed explanations of self-healing techniques and methods of teaching others to heal themselves. Also included are ways to avoid absorbing negative, sick energies from others.

The navel's center is where negative emotions, stress, tension, and sickness accumulate and congest. When this occurs, all vital functions stagnate. Using Chi Nei Tsang techniques in and around the area of the navel provides the fastest method of healing and the most permanent results.

By Master Mantak Chia and Maneewan Chia. Published by Healing Tao Books. Softbound. 448 pages.

$16.95 plus $1.95 for postage & handling
(Foreign Shipping: Please see page Catalog-39)
Order by Item No. B10

FORTHCOMING PUBLICATIONS

- **Awakening Healing Light**—The foundation meditation practice of the Healing Tao System for channeling energy and self-empowerment.
- **Tai Chi Chi Kung I**—The inner structure of Tai Chi.
- **Five Element Nutrition**—Ancient Chinese cooking based on the Five Elements Theory.
- **Fusion of the Five Elements II**—Thrusting and Belt Channels. Growing positive emotions, psychic and emotional self-defense.
- **Cosmic Chi Kung**—Techniques developing healing hands and ability to heal from a distance.

VHS VIDEOS

Invite Master Chia into your living room.

$55.00 per tape. Please order by Item Number. Our videos are not compatible with the PAL System. **Add postage and handling as follows: 1 video—$3.00, 2 videos—$4.75, 3 or more videos—$5.50.** (**Foreign Shipping**: Please see page Catalog-39)

✻ *New From 1992*

Item	Title
V50-TP1	Tai Chi Chi Kung I / Theory and Practice (Vol.1)
V50-TP2	Tai Chi Chi Kung I / Theory and Practice (Vol.2)
✻V51-TP1	Tai Chi Chi Kung II / Theory and Practice (Vol.1)
✻V51-TP2	Tai Chi Chi Kung II / Theory and Practice (Vol.2)
✻V52-TP	Chi Sel Massage/Theory and Practice
✻V58-TP1	Bone Marrow Nei Kung/T&P (Vol. 1)
✻V58-TP2	Bone Marrow Nei Kung/T&P (Vol. 2
V60-TP	Cosmic Chi Kung /T&P(Buddha Palm Advanced)

✻ *New From 1993* —Each volume $39.95

✻V59-TP **Volumes 1—4** Iron Shirt II/Theory & Practice

Weekend Workshops

Item	Title
V57-TP	Iron Shirt Chi Kung I / Theory and Practice
V61-T	Microcosmic Orbit / Theory
V61-M	Microcosmic Orbit / Meditation
V62-TP	Six Healing Sounds / Theory and Practice
V63-T	Healing Love through The Tao / Theory
V63-P	Healing Love through The Tao / Practice
V64-T	Fusion of Five Elements I / Theory
V64-M	Fusion of Five Elements I / Meditation
V65-T	Fusion of Five Elements II / Theory
V65-M	Fusion of Five Elements II / Meditation
V66-T	Fusion of Five Elements III / Theory
V66-M	Fusion of Five Elements III / Meditation
V67-TP1	Chi Nei Tsang / Theory and Practice (Vol.1)
V67-TP2	Chi Nei Tsang / Theory and Practice (Vol.2)
V68-P	Chi Nei Tsang's Healing Power Practice

CASSETTE TAPES

Guided Practice Tapes C09-C18 are guided by Master Mantak Chia.
(Foreign Shipping: Please see page Catalog-39)

Item No.	Title	No. of Tapes	Price	Domestic Postage & Handling
C09	Inner Smile	1	$ 9.95	$ 1.95
C10	Six Healing Sounds	1	9.95	1.95
C11	Microcosmic Orbit	1	9.95	1.95
C11a	Healing Love	1	9.95	1.95
C12	Tai Chi Chi Kung I	1	9.95	1.95
C13	Iron Shirt Chi Kung I	1	9.95	1.95
C14	Sitting Meditation for Home Instruction		9.95	1.95
C15	Standing Meditation for Home Instruction		9.95	1.95
C16	Fusion of the Five Elements I	1	9.95	1.95
C17	Fusion of the Five Elements II	1	9.95	1.95
C18	Fusion of the Five Elements III	1	9.95	1.95

Weekend Workshops
Taught by Master Mantak Chia.

Item No.	Title	No. of Tapes	Price	Domestic Postage & Handling
C19	Microcosmic Orbit: complete the Microcosmic Orbit, Six Healing Sounds, Inner Smile	6	$ 42.00	$ 3.95
C20	Tai Chi Chi Kung I	4	30.00	3.95
C21	Iron Shirt Chi Kung I	4	30.00	3.95
C23	Iron Shirt Chi Kung III	4	30.00	3.95
C24	Fusion of the Five Elements I	4	30.00	3.95
C25	Fusion of the Five Elements II	4	30.00	3.95
C26	Fusion of the Five Elements III	4	30.00	3.95
C27	Healing Love	4	30.00	3.95

CASSETTE TAPES

Retreats (sold only in complete sets)

Item No.	Title	Price	Domestic Postage & Handling
C29	Lesser Kan and Li	$189.00	$6.50
C30	Greater Kan and Li	189.00	6.50
C31	Greatest Kan and Li	189.00	6.50

BONE MARROW NEI KUNG (IRON SHIRT) EQUIPMENT

(**Foreign Shipping**: Please see page Catalog-39)

Item No.	Title	Price	Postage & Handling
62C	Untreated Drilled Jade Egg with Handbook	$15.95	$3.75
62D	Bar for the Chi Weight-Lifting Exercise	15.95	3.75
62E	Wire Hitter (for Bone Marrow Nei Kung)	15.00	3.75
62F	Rattan Hitter (for Bone Marrow Nei Kung)	15.00	3.75
62G	100% Silk Cloth for Chi Weight-Lifting and Massage	10.00	1.95
62H	Partial Set: Vaginal Chi Weight-Lifting Equipment Only (includes 62C, 62D, 62G)	39.95	7.25
62I	Set of Chi Weight-Lifting and Hitting Equipment for Women (includes 62C, 62D, 62E, 62F, 62G and 62K)	75.00	10.00
62J	Set of Chi Weight-Lifting and Hitting Equipment for Men (includes 62D, 62E, 62F, 62G and 62K)	60.00	9.25
62K	Bag (For Equipment)	10.00	1.95

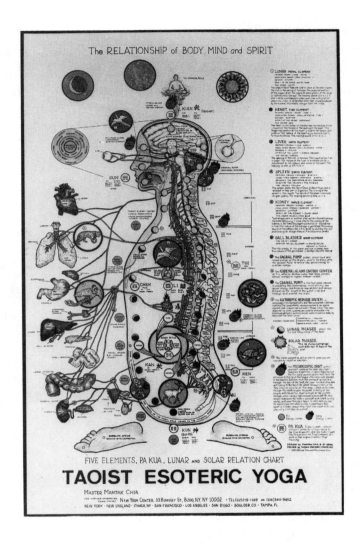

TAO BODY/MIND/SPIRIT CHART 23″ x 35″, full-color chart by Susan McKay.
$7.50 per copy plus $1.95 for postage and handling
(Foreign Shipping: Please see page Catalog-39)
Order by Item No. C H47

POSTERS

18 × 22″, four-color process posters were created by artist Juan Li. Please order by item number.

$7.50 per poster, plus $1.95 for postage and handling.
On orders of three or more posters, $4.60 postage and handling.
$95.00 per set of fourteen posters, free postage and handling.
(Foreign Shipping: Please see page Catalog-39)
Order by Item No. 45.

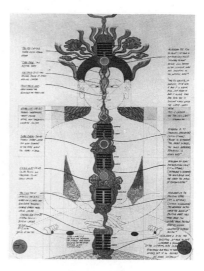

The Microcosmic Orbit—Small Heavenly Cycle—The Functional Channel (Yin).
The Microcosmic Orbit Meditation is the key to circulating internal healing energy, and is the gateway to higher Taoist Meditations.
Item No. P31

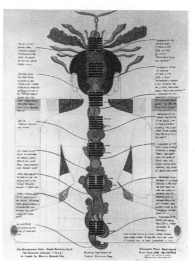

The Microcosmic Orbit—Small Heavenly Cycle—The Governor Channel (Yang).
The Governor Channel of the Microcosmic Orbit Meditation allows the Yang (hot) energy to flow from the base of the spine to the brain.
Item No. P32

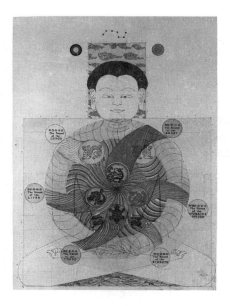

The Six Healing Sounds. The Six Healing Sounds dispel illness, relieve stress, and cool overheated emotions.
Item No. P33

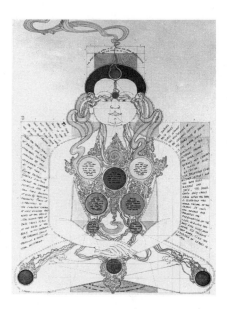

The Secret of the Inner Smile. The Inner Smile is the secret for living in simple harmony with yourself and others. The Inner Smile is the smile of total happiness. This is not the social smile. This smile rises from the cells and organs of the body.
Item No. P34

Healing Love and Sex—Seminal Kung Fu. By conserving their seeds during lovemaking, men can transform sexual energy into spiritual love, and, at the same time, enjoy a higher orgasm. The main purpose of Seminal and Ovarian Kung Fu is to utilize sexual energy for attaining higher levels of consciousness so that the sexual urge does not control the person.
Item No. P35

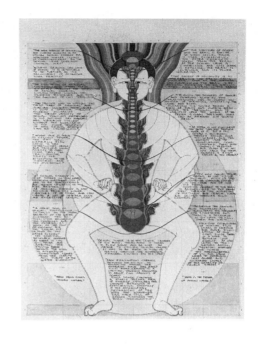

Healing Love and Sex— Ovarian Kung Fu. The Taoists teach women to regulate their menstrual flow and transmute sexual orgasm into higher spiritual love. The techniques of Seminal and Ovarian Kung Fu allow the practitioner to harness sexual impulses so that sex does not control the person. By controlling sexual impulses, people are able to move from the mortal level into higher levels of consciousness. **Item No. P36**

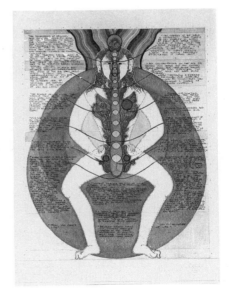

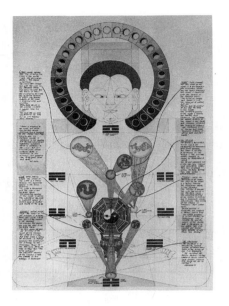

Fusion of the Five Elements I—Cleansing, Clearing, and Harmonizing of the Organs and the Emotions. Each organ stores a separate emotional energy. When fused into a single balanced Chi at the navel, the opening of the six special channels becomes possible.
Item No. P37

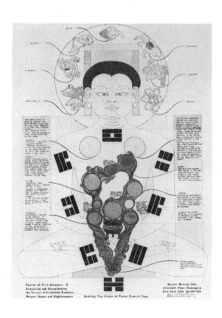

Fusion of the Five Elements II—Enhancing and Strengthening the Virtues. Fusion of the Five Elements II strengthens positive emotions, balances the organs, and encourages in men and women the natural virtues of gentleness, kindness, respect, honor, and righteousness.
Item No. P38

Fusion of the Five Elements II—Thrusting Channels. Running through the center of the body, the Thrusting Routes allow the absorption of cosmic energies for greater radiance and power.
 Item No. P39

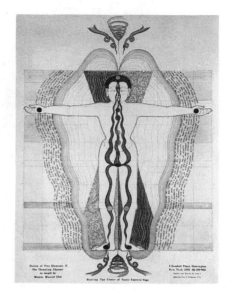

Fusion of the Five Elements II—Nine Belt Channel. The Taoist Belt Channel spins a web of Chi around the major energy vortexes in the body, protecting the psyche by connecting the power of Heaven and Earth.
Item No. P40

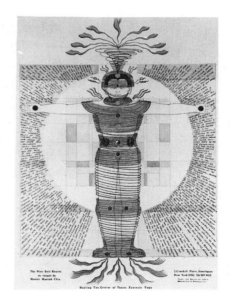

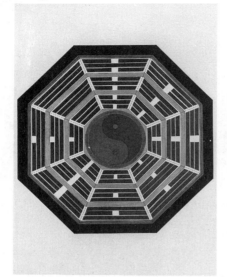

Pa Kua. The Cauldron of Fusing the Energy and Emotions. **Item No. P42**

The Harmony of Yin and Yang. "Yin cannot function without the help of Yang; Yang cannot function without the help of Yin." —Taoist Canon, 8th century A.D. **Item No. P41**

Fusion of the Five Elements III—Yin Bridge and Regulator Channels. Fusion of the Five Elements III uses special meridians to cleanse the aura and regulate high-voltage energy absorbed by the body during meditation. **Item No. P43**

Fusion of the Five Elements III—Yang Bridge and Regulator Channels. Fusion of the Five Elements III teaches the yogic secrets of safely regulating the release of the kundalini power using special meridians. **Item No. P44**

CHI CARD

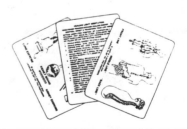

Item No.	Title	Price	Domestic Postage & Handling
CC01	Chi Card - Level 1	9.95	1.95
CC02	Chi Card - Level 2	9.95	1.95

(**Foreign Shipping:** Please see page Catalog-39)

HOW TO ORDER

Prices and Taxes: Subject to change without notice.New York State residents please add 8.5% sales tax.

Payment: Personal check, money order, certified check, or bank cashier's check to: **HEALING TAO BOOKS, INC.**
P.O. BOX 1194
Huntington, NY 11743
Tel. (516) 367 - 2701 — FAX: (516) 367-2754

Mastercard, Visa, and American Express credit cards accepted. **All foreign checks should be International Money Orders or checks drawn on a U.S. bank.**

Domestic Shipping:

Shipping via UPS requires a complete street address . Please include special mailing requests. Allow 3-4 weeks for delivery.
(Foreign Shipping: Please see below)*** .

Special rate products (Domestic Shipping Only):
VHS Video Tapes: 1 Tape--$3.00 2 Tapes--$4.75 3 or More--$5.50
Entire Set of posters - free shipping and handling
All Workshop Cassette Tapes: $3.95 per set
All Kan & Li Cassette Tapes: $6.95 per set

All other products Domestic Shipping and Handling Charges

Order Total	Zone 1-6	Zones 7 & 8
$14.00 or less	$1.95	$1.95
14.01 - 20.00	3.75	3.75
20.01 - 30.00	5.75	5.75
30.01 - 40.00	6.95	7.25
40.01 - 50.00	7.75	8.50
50.01 - 60.00	8.50	9.25
60.01 - 70.00	9.25	10.00
70.01 - 80.00	9.75	10.75
80.01 - 90.00	10.00	11.25
90.01 - 100.00	10.25	11.75
100.01 - 120.00	11.00	13.50
120.01 - 140.00	12.00	14.50
140.01 - 200.00	14.50	19.25
Over 200.00	$3.75/every$50	$4.75/every$50

Zones 7 & 8: Zip codes with the first 3 digits:
577, 586 - 593, 677 - 679, 690, 693
733, 739, 763 - 772, 774 - 774, 778 - 797, 798 - 799
800 - 899, 900 - 994
All other Zip codes are Zones 1 - 6

****Foreign Shipping***: by *surface mail*($5.95 per book), *air mail* ($12.95 per book). *Other products double the domestic rate above for surface mail.* Please call or write for additional information in your area.

THE INTERNATIONAL
HEALING TAO CENTERS

For further information about any of our courses or centers, or to order books, posters, etc., please write or call:

The Healing Tao Center
P.O. Box 1194, Huntington, NY 11743
Phone: (516) 367-2701
Fax: (516) 367-2754

There are also Healing Tao Centers in:

UNITED STATES
- Arizona
- California
  Los Angeles
  San Francisco
- Colorado
- Connecticut
- Delaware
- Florida
- Hawaii
- Illinois
- Massachusetts
- Michigan
- Minnesota
- New Jersey
- New Mexico
- New York
- North Carolina
- Oklahoma
- Oregon
- Pennsylvania
- South Dakota
- Wisconsin

BERMUDA

CANADA
- Ontario
- British Columbia
- Quebec

EUROPE
- Austria
- England
- France
- Greece
- Holland
- Switzerland
- Netherlands
- Spain
- Germany
- Italy

ASIA
- Japan
- India

AUSTRALIA

NOTES

NOTES